SibCare:
The Trip You Never Planned to Take

Caring for a sister or brother with a disability or serious illness can be tricky across distance, competing family priorities, and personalities. *SibCare* is essential in orienting someone who may not know where to start. Its pages are filled with goal-oriented and practical advice: direct, no-nonsense, and useful.

As a professional researcher, sibling organization founder, and sibling of two brothers with disabilities, I wholeheartedly recommend this book.

John Kramer, PhD
Sibling Leadership Network co-founder

Most folks don't expect to care for a sibling with medical problems. Most folks don't even think about it. Then, **Bam!** Your life is suddenly interrupted by a brother's or sister's health crisis.

Sibling relationships are usually the longest of your entire life. Your parents are there at the beginning. A partner and children may join you for the middle and later years. But the sibs are generally along for the entire journey, marching with you side by side through your family's history.

SibCare: The Trip You Never Planned to Take
is your road map when that family journey detours into medical terrain.

www.SibCare.org

SibCare
The Trip You Never Planned to Take

TAFFY CANNON

BLUE SKIES PRESS

USA

© Taffy Cannon, 2016

Published by Blue Skies Press.

ISBN: **978-0-9978053-0-7**

For permissions and more information please visit

www.sibcare.org

or write to

Blue Skies Press
PO Box 2520
Carlsbad CA 92018

SibCare: The Trip You Never Planned to Take, by Taffy Cannon.

ISBN: 978-0-9978053-0-7

1. Family 2. Siblings 3. Home health care 4. Resources for Caregivers 5.Title

Sib**Care**

TABLE OF CONTENTS

• • • • •

Note: Additional resources are included at
the end of each topic.

INTRODUCTION

I never wanted to write this book.

I never wanted to learn—often haphazardly and on the fly—the information included here. But when I needed that information, I couldn't find it. This is the book I wanted when my own family faced the issue of SibCare, head-on and clueless.

If you've gotten this far, you probably have a sister or brother with serious medical issues, quite possibly living some distance away. You may even *be* that sibling, wondering how you are going to manage a blizzard of unfamiliar situations and options as you move into new and frightening medical territory.

Odds are good in either case that you have managed your own life pretty well and weren't expecting this detour at this point, or maybe ever. Also that you're some combination of nervous, angry, confused, scared, lonely, and weary.

You've got a lot of company.

Because the reality is that when your health turns on you, if you don't have a good support system already in place, the default is always going to be family.

Serious sibling illness can occur at any age, and is generally awful. It is now beginning to strike with some regularity among baby boomers who are getting old. I know that because I'm one of them.

The generation that was going to stay Forever Young has had a pretty good shot at it, and many of us have worked very hard at remaining youthful. However, the oldest baby boomers are already on Medicare and Social Security, and others are looking at various retirement scenarios, while carefully avoiding thinking about the end of the trail.

Unfortunately, the end of the trail sometimes jumps up and slaps you on the butt.

For my family, that slap came in January 2008 when my sister and brother and I began a journey we didn't want to take, on an unmapped road through mine fields that none of us had ever considered before.

We made mistakes and followed false paths and spent a lot of time with our fingers in our ears, singing *lalalalalalalala* very loudly. We learned to live by a maxim our mother used often: "We'll cross that bridge when we get to it."

Our family journey ended four years later on March 12, 2012, when my brother died at the age of 54.

We weren't particularly close when all this began, though nobody was seriously estranged. Our mother had died in 1971 and our father in 1993. We spoke occasionally and visited infrequently, usually around some event unrelated to family. In that sense we were like a lot of families that scattered in the seventies, when baby boomers often headed out in interesting directions and never came back.

Now we crashed into a fundamental reality: When you're on your own without a strong local support system and your health turns on you, the default is family. Wherever they may be and wherever you may be.

In our family, I was the oldest, my sister Chris four years younger, and our brother Bill four years younger still. When everything started, I lived in San Diego, Chris in Seattle, and Bill in the western suburbs of Chicago. When it ended, the only address that had changed was Bill's, though he still lived in Illinois.

Bill was 51 in 2008, a long-term malignant brain tumor survivor, a divorced former cop now working as a booking clerk at the county jail. Fourteen years after his brain tumor saga began, he was living alone and the tumor had never returned.

Chris and I knew that since his original treatment in

1994 he'd experienced some whopping seizures that often required hospitalization, but we both considered his health stable and he pretty much ignored it altogether. There were signs that his overall condition was deteriorating, but we hadn't acted—or known how to act—on those signs. The tumor had never returned, after all, and that was what we'd all been quietly expecting and dreading.

Then the Cannon Family Parade of Holidays began, a phenomenon we might have submitted to Ripley's if only we could find the time.

Nearly all the strokes and seizures over the coming four years were tied to major national holidays. I grew to approach three-day weekends with dread and was known to celebrate when it got to be Tuesday without a call from the ER.

Each medical event brought additional brain damage and more memory problems in somebody who was, from the neck down, otherwise in excellent physical condition. I made a lot of trips back to the Midwest, often in inauspicious weather.

By the time our Parade of Holidays ended—five days shy of St. Patrick's Day—my sister and I had dealt with an entire decathlon of SibCare problems and issues:

1. Ongoing physical and mental deterioration of somebody we really loved
2. Financial issues with everybody from the local hardware store to the IRS
3. Property with half-finished renovation projects that needed to be cleared, listed, and sold, in a stagnant market
4. Insurance companies, banks, medical facilities, and governmental bureaucracies of all sizes
5. A wide range of medical specialists in multiple locations
6. Continually changing but never entirely effective medications
7. The need to separate a middle-aged man from his beloved truck and the house he adored, permanently
8. Four different downsizing operations, culminating in a single large room of an assisted living facility

9. The extraordinary good fortune and karma of having a family who loved him step up as caregivers
10. All of the above occurring long distance, some 1800 miles away from either of his sisters.

My sister and I were running blind most of the time, dealing with situations as they arose and hoping for the best. We made mistakes. We got lucky more than once. We learned not to look too far down the road, because whenever we tried to plan ahead, we hit a sinkhole.

There were periods when I felt my entire life was being consumed by my brother's medical melodrama. There were also times when I went merrily about my own business and only rarely thought of Bill, mostly when I paid his bills or talked to Chris, who spoke with him frequently.

As we stumbled through this uncharted territory, I realized only dimly that we were inventing SibCare as we went along, long distance and on the fly. I was never entirely certain what might be coming next, other than another holiday which might find my brother arriving at the Emergency Room by ambulance, in *status epileptus.*

When I think about it in those terms now, I marvel that we ever got anything done, much less done right.

He was a hell of a guy, my brother, and I loved him dearly, but caring for him was often frustrating and complicated, and doing it all long distance proved to be a gargantuan challenge.

It would have been easier with a guidebook, and that's what this book is about. So that when you find yourself suddenly flailing about in the quagmire of SibCare, you have somewhere to start. There's a lot of information here, and a wealth of additional resources for areas that you may need to explore in depth.

Nobody needs to read or learn it all.

With luck there will be huge areas that you can skip altogether because they're not an issue for your family. In many cases, your own family medical situation may be so specialized that you can only use specific resources listed here as jumping-off points.

This book isn't intended to be all-inclusive, but my goal is to point you in the right directions and give you the tools and general information you need to head off along those paths with your sibling at your side. And if one or the other of you happens to be grumbling at any given moment on that journey, wasn't it always kind of like that?

My brother was a hippie, a Marine, a cop, a brain tumor survivor, a gardener, a war gamer, a gourmet cook, and a silver-tongued Irishman with a quick temper and a quicker grin. He was smart and clever and quick and funny and creative.

He fought long and hard, sometimes against all reason and through sheer pigheadedness. Life dealt him a really crummy hand, but he played it with dignity and honor. He never lost his optimism, though he grew stoic about what happened to him and his brain.

He loved being a cop, and one of his oft-expressed laments was, "All I ever wanted to do was help people."

He still is.

I dedicate this book to Bill Cannon, with confidence that what our family learned together will help others traverse the perilous rope bridge of SibCare.

Love you, Baby Brother.

SECTION ONE:

WARMING UP

THIS IS NOT LIKE TAKING CARE OF YOUR PARENTS

Caring for an aging parent and caring for an ailing sibling share certain common ground.

The cast of characters is much the same, illness is generally involved, and the person being helped may not want assistance. It may be necessary to physically relocate somebody, and that somebody might not want to go. Unless you are unbelievably rich, money invariably figures into matters, particularly related to health care expenses. And when paid caregiving gets added to the equation, dollar signs fly through the air as if you'd stumbled onto the soundstage of a Thirties musical.

However.

Your siblings are not your parents. The relationships you've had with your siblings are all different, and roughly on the same latitude. While you were growing up, your parents took care of all of you, because that was their responsibility. You and your siblings, if you were lucky, took care of each other.

The relationships with your brothers and sisters are likely to be the longest ones you'll have in your entire life. Your parents are there for the first part, a partner and children may be around for the middle and final parts, but the sibs are mostly along for the entire journey, marching with you side by side through your family's history.

Yes, many families are dysfunctional, some supremely so. But over time you have probably developed coping mechanisms that will help you accommodate your family's particular version of dysfunction now, when you really *do* need to work together.

THE NATURAL ORDER OF THINGS

One important distinction between caring for parents and siblings is that taking responsibility for aging parents is a cultural expectation for most of us.

Until actually thrust into a SibCare situation, however, most of us haven't given a moment's thought to caring for siblings. And why would we? In some internal photo album, we carry around snapshots of our siblings when we were all kids—healthy and active and foolhardy, ready to take on the world. And that's often how we still see each other, even when irrefutable evidence shows a very different picture.

You may have grown up with grandparents who moved in at some point, or maybe were always there. If the grandparents moved in early enough, there was often a transitional period where they helped out with the kids. It all seemed perfectly natural, whether the experiment in cohabitation worked or not. My mother's father moved in with us when I was in fifth grade and my father's mother moved in with my cousins a few years later. Nobody ever thought a thing about it, though I wouldn't describe either situation as a glowing success.

It was a social contract: Your parents helped you and later you helped them. Period.

Two things have happened to this stereotype in recent decades.

First, as the Greatest Generation aged, they often didn't *want* to move in with their children, or even to have their children nearby. Having survived the Great Depression and World War II, they were determined to remain as independent as they possibly could for as long as they possibly could.

They were generally pretty good at it, too. A whole new world of multi-level retirement communities arose, places where seniors could move from their own self-contained apartments to assisted living to a nursing home—without ever having to leave the mother ship.

Secondly, their children were often a little too busy to even consider having Mom and/or Dad move in, what with juggling two jobs and sports transport and scouts and games and dance and parent conferences while trying to steal the occasional free moment for themselves.

However, the expectation of parental care remains so deeply ingrained in both our society and personal upbringing that it's probably in our DNA as well by now. And it isn't limited to homo sapiens, either.

A few years ago, we got a pound kitten when our elderly cat Jezebel was clearly in her final illness, taking daily medication and suffering a form of kitty dementia. The intention was to provide a kind of transitional buffer zone, but the reality surprised us all. Rebecca attached herself to Jezebel as a sort of round-the-clock special duty nurse: attending her, grooming her, following her around to keep her safe.

Indeed, she set such a high standard of care that it was something of a relief to realize that our own parents were long gone and would not require the same level of attention.

ONGOING CONTACT

In general, children of all ages remain in some contact with their parents.

This contact may not be daily or weekly or even monthly. It may not involve regular dinners or shopping excursions or joint vacations or even celebration of major holidays together, though it usually does include awkward long distance holiday conversations.

Still, folks generally know where their parents are and

how to get in touch with them. This is such a cultural given that during a brief period in my gypsy past when I realized that my father didn't have my address and might not even be aware I was in California, I felt guilty about it. Liberated, but guilty.

The sibling situation can be very different, however, particularly if there have been major issues or problems over time. Estrangement may be the exception, but it happens. And even when sibs aren't formally estranged, they may be scattered hither and yon with only occasional and random communication among themselves.

UNRESOLVED ISSUES

It's entirely possible to have unresolved (and unresolvable) issues with parents, even when the combined parent and child ages total over 150 years. But as time passes, these issues may become inactive. They're either set aside or you figure out a way to work around them. Dementia may also be a factor with parents, a cruel and double-edged sword that pretty much eliminates the potential for resolution and reconciliation.

Sibling issues, however, often feel more fresh. And for those who resolved differences by hitting the road and never looking back, they can be frozen in time. It may seem silly to remain mad at your brother forty years after he didn't come to your first wedding but grudges are sustained over far less.

NOT EVERYBODY GETS INVOLVED IN PARENTAL CARE

Some parents die young and often those deaths are sudden and unexpected.

I had just turned 23 when my 50-year-old mother died of a cerebral aneurysm that burst in the course of a normal afternoon and killed her less than 24 hours later. It was fast, it was horrible, it was unfair—but it happened. My husband's mother died of cancer when she was 46. Even back then it seemed they were far too young to die, and realizing that my mother has missed two-thirds of my life is an ongoing sorrow.

But losing our mothers when they were so very young has given me a different perspective on many things, including the griping of my friends about the demands of their own aging moms. I would gladly trade some of that aggravation to have had the opportunity for my mother and daughter to know each other.

A second wave of parents generally dies in their sixties and seventies, often of cancer or heart attacks. In many of those situations, which generally aren't as abrupt, final care comes from the other parent or a step-parent, in scenarios that involve limited participation by any children, much less all of them. There might be a final visit, and almost always a church service with food back at the house, but if you aren't living in town, you usually aren't as actively involved.

Then there are the parents who are truly old—octogenarian and nonagenarian and even centenarian. But the reality is that there actually aren't all that many of them. We simply hear so much from the people who care for super-senior parents that it just *seems* like everybody is doing it.

The lines are drawn differently with sibling care, and offer far less clarity. If you're all around the same age, there's no telling who might get sick, or need back surgery, or have some unexpected and unpleasant medical surprise. It can happen to pretty much anybody who has a sister or a brother.

You might even be the patient yourself.

DIFFERENT LEVELS OF EXPECTATION

Society is pretty clear on this one.

If you have a parent in need of help, you're expected to come through. This is the person who paced and held you while you screamed during sleepless nights of colic. Who baked brownies for the school bake sale, found your missing mitten, taught you how to make a slow pitch, and waited anxiously for the sound of the garage door when you first hit the road with a newly-issued driver's license.

When it's your turn, you either step up or you're

awarded a big fat societal black eye.

A sibling, however, is another matter entirely. If you are inclined to walk away from a sibling illness, you might not appear to be the world's kindest person, but people won't automatically recoil in horror. Anyone with siblings will understand that these can be problematic relationships.

So you're more likely to get a pass, which makes it easier to walk away with minimal, or at least lessened, guilt.

THE POSSIBILITY OF RECOVERY

When you assume responsibility for a parent's care, you know that somewhere down the line, that responsibility will end and your parent will die, most likely before you do. Cold, but true.

Not so with siblings.

It's entirely possible that your ailing sibling will make a full and complete recovery from the physical problem at the heart of your current relationship. It may in fact be your participation that helps make that recovery possible.

Rewards come in strange ways at strange times.

ADULT SIBLING RELATIONSHIPS

I don't believe an accident of birth makes people sisters or brothers. It makes them siblings, gives them mutuality of parentage. Sisterhood and brotherhood is a condition people have to work at.

Maya Angelou

Perhaps the most interesting thing about the study of adult sibling relationships is that there is so little of it.

In a world where every possible relationship has been analyzed, scrutinized, and dissected, this most fundamental link has been all but ignored. In fact, the most attention has been given to the element over which an individual has the least control: birth order.

BIRTH ORDER

The notion that birth order plays a significant role was first publicly promulgated in the early 20th Century by Alfred Adler, the Austrian physician who also gave us the notion of the inferiority complex. Adler, the second of seven children, suffered from severe rickets and considered his older brother the family star. He asserted that the second child in a family had ambition, competitiveness, and a desire to best the older sibling.

Since Adler first wrote about this in 1928, birth order theory has surfaced with some regularity and has woven itself into pop culture expectations. It makes good introductory chatter (certainly better than "What's your sign?") and can adjust to fit almost any situation.

At its most stripped down, birth order theory works

roughly like this:

First-borns are princes and princesses, who have the advantage of undivided parental attention in their earliest years and are likely to be high achievers.

Middle children have to fight for attention and are likely to be independent, loyal, and diplomatic chameleons.

The baby of the family tends to be charming, fun, easygoing, and comfortable seeking and holding attention—with a manipulative streak when necessary.

All three descriptions focus on attention, which is often the primary currency of childhood, whether from parents, siblings, neighbors, babysitters, teachers, relatives, or friends. Anybody who believes in birth order theory can list famous examples for each category.

But it really isn't that simple. There are indeed a disproportionate number of first-born presidents, scientists, Nobel Laureates, and captains of industry. However, a 1970 Swiss study also found a disproportionate number of first-born strippers (90%!) and unwed mothers. Fact is, this is the kind of thing you can twist any way you want. Charlie Manson, Ted Bundy, and Jeffrey Dahmer were also first-borns. So there.

The reality is that endless variables determine personality traits and family dynamics and are at least as significant as birth order. Economic status, gender, school history, illness, intervals between children, divorce, and other family disruptions—pretty much anything but the phase of the moon can factor in. Maybe the phase of the moon does, too.

GENETICS

Still, if the members of a family all start out in the same gene pool, you'd expect to find more similarities than actually exist. Despite many family units with peas-in-a-pod children, others feature siblings with nothing apparent in common except an address and a couple who claim to have sired and birthed them.

A very dumbed-down mini-seminar on genetics can partially explain this. When sperm and egg come together, each of them carries a full set of chromosomes. These two sets need to be merged into one single full set. While nobody entirely understands how these chromosome v. chromosome decisions are made (Rock, paper, scissors? Seductive charm? Physical force?) we do know that only one of each pair will dominate in every genetic face-off.

This suggests a 50-50 split on genetic characteristics, but the actual range is between 35 percent and 65 percent, which also explains why some sibling pairs so seem more alike than others.

Robert Plomin of the Institute of Psychiatry at the University of London maintains that sibling similarities are most likely due to common genes, while differences arise equally from genetics and childhood environment. But while kids may *seem* to have the same childhood environment, this is only true in the kind of horrible orphan warehouses where babies lie in their own waste in rows of identical cribs.

Your experiences growing up were different from the other kids on the block and they weren't precisely the same ones that your brothers and sisters had growing up in the same household, either. Even identical twins have similar but different lives.

Dalton Conley in *The Pecking Order* claims convincingly that all sorts of external factors come into play for any sibling relationship: physical distance between siblings, spacing of siblings, parental economic status at various stages of family life, school history, illness—in short, the entire universe outside of that initial egg and sperm.

Nature versus nurture remains a very real question, short on definitive answers.

OTHER ADULT SIBLING ISSUES

I read a lot of books about adult siblings, picked up some interesting trivia (Anna Freud had to give up the piano because her practicing disturbed older brother Sigmund, for instance) and realized pretty quickly that nobody was writing about assuming care for an ailing adult sibling. I soldiered on anyway, looking for answers. Explanations. *Something.*

In *Original Kin: The Search for Connection Among Adult Sisters and Brothers,* Marian Sandmaier reviewed psychological research on siblings from the mid-1980s through the mid-1990s and found 98 studies about birth order, 185 about the effect of a chronically ill or disabled sibling, 65 about the death of a sibling in childhood and 34 on gender. Not much seems to have changed since then.

Sandmaier also speaks of "turning points" in sibling relationships that can alter everything forever. A surprising 85% of adults aged 22-93 recalled a specific incident which improved or worsened a relationship with a sibling. This event can occur at any age, and these turning points can move a sibling relationship in all sorts of different directions.

Sometimes forever.

The study of the most relevance to the topic of SibCare was conducted by Deborah Gold of Duke University on types of adult sibling relationships. As you look through the following list, it's impossible not to see your own relationships on it. Many different configurations are possible within a single family, too. Every sibling has a specific relationship with every other sibling and they're all different. Gold divided them in this fashion:

17% Intimate
28% Congenial
35% Loyal
10% Apathetic
10% Hostile

It's usually pretty easy to figure out how your own siblings fit these categories.

The lines may blur a bit between Intimate and Congenial, or between Congenial and Loyal. But it's pretty hard to mistake Hostile for anything else, and you can probably already hear your Apathetic sib heave a mighty sigh and mutter "whatever" when informed that your brother contracted a rare paralytic infection while hang-gliding in the Amazon basin and isn't expected to see his next birthday.

Recognizing how these relationships are constructed in

your own family and how they vary from one sibling to another can help you better approach others for specific or general help. Just don't assume that because your relationship to your brother is Loyal, so is your sister's. She may consider it Intimate because he once helped her out of a jam that nobody but the two of them knows about, or Hostile because he refused to do so. And he might be Apathetic to you both.

You are also likely to discover significant gender differences. Most libraries and bookstores feature groaning shelves on the problems that men and women have relating to one another, whether or not they happen to be kinfolk. There's no need for a lengthy discussion here of how guys are more likely to talk about next Saturday's game while gals want to get into their feelings. But it's worth noting that when psychologist Deborah Tannen took on sibling relationships in *You Were Always Mom's Favorite,* the focus was on sisters and not brothers.

Sibling relationships can and do change over time, and nowhere is this more likely to occur than under the pressure of a family medical crisis. Everything may upend itself repeatedly, too. You may find yourself allied with somebody who formerly had very little to do with you, or ready to throttle somebody who once seemed totally simpatico.

Until a new round of Medical Chairs begins and everybody shifts positions again.

"BABY, WE WERE BORN TO RUN"

Gold notes that people with higher educational levels and social standing are less likely to be involved with their siblings later in life. This may be because these higher achievers have wider social networks and can seek help from non-family members, though a sudden sibling health crisis can blow a giant ragged hole in that scenario.

For the baby boomers and the generations that have followed, one variable not examined nearly enough is the fluidity and flexibility of youth. Many wind up settling somewhere far from home, perhaps offering a quiet sigh of relief at the same time.

Often that works out pretty well for everybody.

Here's the rub: If one of the reasons why somebody went away and never came back was issues with other family members, those issues probably didn't fix themselves in their absence. They remained behind, quietly festering.

Does this matter? Maybe not. Sometimes time really does resolve this stuff and everybody embraces tearfully and promises never to be so silly again.

But when folks have been hanging on to bad feelings or memories for a long time, it's rarely quite so simple and may need to be addressed. Go back to the simple question: What happened? If you ask two siblings who have remained annoyed with each other for years to explain what created the rift, it is possible that both recall the incident with excruciating, blame-ridden details that are entirely different. You get responses not unlike that group of blind people describing an elephant based on whether they were touching an ear, trunk, leg, or tail.

Meanwhile, the emotions remain white-hot.

A lot comes down to simple common sense, as put forth by Susan Scharf Merrell in *The Accidental Bond: The Power of Sibling Relationships.* Merrell offers five steps toward improving a sibling relationship, first noting that before a difficult relationship can be fixed, it's necessary to make a conscious decision to do so. If you can get that far, she suggests:

1. Put the past in the past.
2. Be honest but not hurtful.
3. Accept your sibling for who she has become.
4. Try to connect with siblings the way you do with friends, on common ground.
5. Don't ask for trouble.

If you just can't bring yourself to do all that, recognize that it won't hurt anything to at least take a stab at part of it.

Best not to make that stab literal, of course.

• • • • •

ADDITIONAL INFORMATION

Stephen P. Bank and Michael D. Kahn
The Sibling Bond
Basic Books, 1982

Dalton Conley
The Pecking Order: A Bold New Look at How Family and Society Determine Who We Become
Vintage, 2004

Judy Dunn and Robert Plomin
Separate Lives: Why Siblings Are So Different
Basic Books, 1990

Adele Faber and Elaine Mazlish
Between Brothers and Sisters: A Celebration of Life's Most Enduring Relationship
Avon Books, 1989

Peter Goldenthal
Why Can't We Get Along? Healing Adult Sibling Relationships
John Wiley & Sons, 2002

William and Mada Hapworth and Joan Rattner Heilman
Mom Loved You the Best: Understanding Rivalry and Enriching Your Adult Sibling Relationships
Penguin, 1993

Jeffery Kluger
The Sibling Effect: What the Bonds Between Brothers and Sisters Reveal About Us
Riverhead Books, 2011

Kevin Leman
The First-Born Advantage
Revell, 2008

Kevin Leman
The New Birth Order Book: Why You Are the Way You Are
Revell, 1998

Jo Ann Levitt, Marjory Levitt, and Joel Levitt
Sibling Revelry: 8 Steps to Successful Adult Sibling Relationships
Dell Trade, 2001

Patti McDermott
Sisters and Brothers: Resolving Your Adult Sibling Relationships
Lowell House, 1994

Susan Scarf Merrell
The Accidental Bond: The Power of Sibling Relationships
Times Books, 1995

Francine Russo
They're <u>Your</u> Parents, Too! How Siblings Can Survive Their Parents' Aging Without Driving Each Other Crazy
Bantam Books, 2010

Marian Sandmaier
Original Kin: The Search for Connection Among Adult Sisters and Brothers
Plume, 1994

Frank J. Sulloway
Born to Rebel: Birth Order, Family Dynamics, and Creative Lives
Vintage, 1997

Deborah Tannen
You Were Always Mom's Favorite! Sisters in Conversation Throughout Their Lives
Random House, 2009

SECTION TWO:

FIRST THINGS FIRST

GETTING STARTED

A bear that's going to go everywhere
has to start by going somewhere.

This was a favorite line from one of my Little Golden Books when I was very small, and if I remember that little bear's dilemma correctly, he had so many places to go and so many things to do that he couldn't get started on anything.

It often feels like that when you are first immersed in—or, more likely, dumped into—a SibCare situation. And if you have been plunged into a full-blown SibCare crisis, you may feel overwhelmed to the point of paralysis.

Here's the key: **You don't have to do everything and you don't have to do it all right this minute.**

FIGURE OUT WHAT'S HAPPENING

This may seem straightforward. It may even *be* straightforward if you and your sibling are close and have been in frequent contact, discussing medical problems.

Just keep in mind that even if you have been in on the whole sorry mess from the beginning, you may not always have been paying full attention. Indeed, there's a good chance you've already inadvertently missed something important.

Matters are even more complicated if you've been out of touch. You are likely to be clueless on many fronts. You may not know much about your sibling's personal life, work situation, health care coverage, general health, financial stability, or spiritual beliefs. Some of these can wait, some are probably urgent, and with a little bit of luck, you won't have to get deeply involved in others.

When my sister and I were thrust into our own SibCare adventure, our younger brother was a 6'2", 200-pound, former cop who had been dealing with significant after-effects of successful brain tumor treatment for fourteen years. He was also smart and cagey and recognized that these continuing problems (which included grand mal seizures) had the potential to jeopardize his job and independence. He enhanced his imposing, get-out-of-my-face persona by shaving his head, and if you happened to notice that revealed a rather nasty scar above his left ear, he didn't mind that either.

What he *hadn't* been doing was sharing information about his medical condition or much of anything else with his sisters, particularly after we staged a thoroughly unsuccessful attempt at a long-distance intervention a few months before his first stroke. And he was so taciturn with coworkers at the county jail where he booked incoming guests that they didn't even know he *had* sisters, though they were aware of his medical problems.

The first stroke changed all that. There was no denying a serious medical condition with major cognitive elements, and most of the landscape was littered with uncertainty.

I was able to accumulate a fair amount of information about the events leading up to my brother's stroke by listening to his coworkers and neighbors, even though he had been generally reticent with all of them. I had an advantage here in that the quality of their observations was unusually high. His only remaining neighborhood buddy was a fellow cop and his coworkers were part of law enforcement. The information they *were* able to offer was sketchy, but precisely because it was so limited, every little bit was important.

HAVE A CONVERSATION

Talk to your brother. Even more important, *listen.* And if he clams up and reaches for the remote, resist the impulse to throttle him, even if that's how the two of you generally have resolved disputes.

Be prepared with a list of questions so you won't forget something and have to bring it up again later. Apologize for invading his privacy and make sure he understands that you wish none of this were happening. Make notes, and if he's uncomfortable about that, explain that it's so you won't need to ask again, ever.

Don't be judgmental about anything. "I told you so" has no part in this conversation.

If your discussion goes down a side alley, follow it until you recognize a clear dead end. Gently rein in somebody who's going too far astray. And if you know that your brother tires easily, keep focusing him forward to cover as much ground as possible before he fades out.

Have him go back to the beginning. Try to find out what—if anything—led up to the current problem. Was it truly a bolt from the blue?

DON'T TAKE ANYTHING FOR GRANTED

Keep in mind that your sibling and others **may or may not have the facts straight.**

When you're sick and in a medical office or hospital room, you don't always hear things accurately. Important information may sail past as you grapple with the shock of what you just heard. Then when you tell family members, you may inadvertently leave out additional key elements because your anxiety is cresting at tsunami levels.

The wonder is that any particulars at all come through correctly. It's like a grown-up version of the childhood game "Telephone" except that the consequences are far more serious if you get the story wrong.

If you think this may be the case, don't challenge what your sister says right away, even if that's your normal style. You may think you're being solicitous and thorough, while she simply finds you overbearing. Take your time and do your own research, or deputize somebody you trust to do it for you.

If you learn things that raise questions that she didn't address, or reveal treatment possibilities that never came up, present this information in a positive and helpful fashion. Even if you're gritting your teeth every second. *Hey, I think I found something promising!* is a lot more effective than *How could you have been so dumb that you missed this?*

WHAT YOU WANT TO FIND OUT

Were there symptoms that your sibling chose to ignore, or did the stroke/heart attack/as-yet-unexplained collapse actually occur without warning? Were there witnesses to the event? Was 911 called? Did your brother ride the ambulance with paramedics performing CPR? Was he admitted through the ER? Any emergency surgery involved? ICU time?

Is there a diagnosis?

This is a biggie. A diagnosis isn't always a given and it isn't even always right. Waiting for it can be hell. But once you *have* a diagnosis, everything moves onto new planes and into new stages.

If there is a diagnosis, what has your sibling been told about it? Pay attention here, but don't assume that his information is absolutely correct, or even mostly correct.

DO YOUR RESEARCH

You need to learn as quickly as possible about the

specific nature of what ails your sibling.

You may already have some of this knowledge. You may have experienced the same problem yourself, know somebody who did, or be aware of a strong family history. There's also a good chance that you never heard about Wellington's Wallop until your brother called to announce his diagnosis.

Once you have some idea of what the medical problem is—however vague that idea might be—start developing your own information sources. Education will become your close personal friend throughout this entire experience.

The critical thing to remember in the beginning is that you don't have to know everything immediately or become the world authority on Wellington's Wallop. All you need to get started is the nature of the immediate problem and how it is being addressed.

Start by plugging "Wellington's Wallop" into a search engine and look for a foundation with a toll-free number. That number will be answered by somebody who knows about the disease, customary treatments, local support groups, and all kinds of things you haven't even had time to think about.

You can even do some of this research during the nail-biting period when there isn't yet a definitive diagnosis but you know you're dealing with a problem related to a particular organ system.

WRITE THINGS DOWN

Keep in mind that in the early stages of any medical situation or crisis, information is the primary currency.

A lot of people go into white coat amnesia after visiting an Emergency Room or doctor's office. Sometimes they're so stunned by one part of what the doctor is saying that they don't even hear the rest.

If it's bad news, you're even more likely to lose memory function. And if you weren't already making notes, you sure aren't going to start slapping pockets looking for a pen and some scratch paper after you hear the word "cancer."

Information that isn't written down can sail off into the sunset with nobody the wiser. In a serious medical situation, this can also cost you time. If you are just coming into the medical scene, see if you can actually look at something official that has the diagnosis on it in words, not medical mumbo jumbo or billing codes. Then start asking questions.

What treatment has been proposed? When would this treatment begin? Have other options been discussed?

Is there a second opinion? Maybe even a third?

NOTIFY PEOPLE

What you need to do and how fast it has to happen mostly has to do with the nature of the situation you're in. If somebody is in ICU with a sudden and shocking prognosis, time matters. If a lifelong jock is getting a knee replaced, there's a lot less urgency.

Start with the obvious family and extended family members. If your sibling doesn't want people to know, respect that, though you may gently argue the case for shared information. Friends and neighbors may already know, particularly if an ambulance was involved.

Keep details off social media unless you have specific permission to post information and even then you should be *very* discreet. Your customary level of sharing information might differ significantly from your sibling's, and you are not the one whose private information is being put onto the Internet, forever.

WIDEN THE CIRCLE OF INQUIRY

While you're clarifying the problem at hand, be sure to also widen the circle of inquiry.

Neighbors, coworkers, and friends of your brother's may have observed something that worried them. Maybe they didn't say anything to him. Maybe they did and he brushed them off. Now is the time to find out whatever you can from whoever's been around.

You're essentially looking for witness statements here, so follow up just like your favorite television detectives would. And don't forget other members of your sib's immediate and extended families, who may have been holding their breath with a sense of doom, waiting for the axe to fall.

The people you come in contact with on your sibling's behalf are likely to be concerned, whether on a personal or a medical level. (Trust me: The unconcerned will either never show up or will disappear quickly.) Be as low-key as you can with friends and coworkers so they'll be more comfortable sharing their concerns and memories with you.

As you exchange information with your sibling's friends, you may feel as if you're talking about two entirely different people, because these people know your brother differently than you do. That's actually good news, particularly if family members have been distanced by miles or emotions or unfortunate episodes of shared history. If you can nail down somebody on the scene who's been paying attention and keeping track, you get to take a giant leap forward on the information-gathering curve. Maybe even over the hump.

Keep in mind that friends don't trash friends.

If you approach your brother's buddies by saying what an idiot he was for never getting any exercise and drinking too much and subsisting on deep-fried everything, they're not going to like it. Nor will they be inclined to cooperate with you. They will more likely leap to his defense and think you are an unsympathetic jerk to be kicking him when he's down.

Being judgmental with your sibling's friends is no better than being judgmental with your sib.

MAKE SHORT-TERM ARRANGEMENTS

The nature of what needs to be done will change with time, and in the beginning those changes can occur quickly. Don't try to plan too far down the road until you know what road you are actually on and where it is going. If you are a planner by nature, this can be hard.

Pay attention to who's offering help, write down names and contact info, and press folks into service right away if you can use them. Be specific with requests because usually people have no idea what is needed or how to help. (You may be one of those people, at least for a while.) Do you need airport pickups, rides to treatment, meal deliveries, or somebody to mow the lawn or shovel the driveway? Try to match talents and availability.

Be flexible, and if something isn't working, or didn't turn out to be as important as you first thought, feel free to make changes.

And don't think you can do everything yourself. You can't.

CAREGIVING CIRCLE
SUPPORT GROUPS

In olden times when someone became ill, neighbors and friends would rally around to assist. Casseroles would be baked, cows milked, children watched after school. Most of us live in a more complicated world, but the same concept has been updated and digitized for the 21st Century. It's a terrific one, discussed in greater depth in the "Caregiving" chapter.

If somebody on your care team wants to create a personal website for your family, that's great, but some very nice people at Caringbridge.org and CarePages.com already have free templates in place for that very purpose. All you need to do is register and start filling in blanks.

These sites are interactive, so well-wishers may post greetings and words of encouragement to both the patient and the patient's family while they keep up with medical developments. (For those who have no idea what to say to somebody in a serious medical situation, suggestions are offered.) You don't have to worry about missing calls or tracking time zones or having a crucial relative three steps behind everybody else's information because a branch snapped off the telephone tree.

Once somebody is given the keys to your own little

web kingdom, it's their responsibility to keep up.

Privacy levels are set by the person who establishes the site and are of extreme importance to the websites themselves. You are, after all, putting confidential personal and medical information into the most public of all media, the Internet. They will work with you to make your sibling's information as readily available or totally inaccessible as your family wishes. If you're holding fundraisers to get your brother a wheelchair-accessible van, you'll set the bar much lower than if your fanatically private sister is battling lung cancer.

RESPECT THE PATIENT

This is absolutely critical.

Your new mantra is: **This is not my illness.**

If your sibling has strong feelings about what should and shouldn't be happening, pay attention. If what he wants is totally unrealistic or maybe even impossible, try to bring him down gently. But work with him to reach decisions that are reasonable.

Nobody likes a bully.

Sick people particularly hate them. They're already experiencing a sense of bewildering helplessness, caught in fast-rushing waters through nasty medical rapids. So be as gentle and caring as possible.

But if reason doesn't enter into your sibling's thought processes at the moment, try to figure out ways to work around him for the time being if necessary. Making progress is not always synonymous with keeping the peace.

It may be that your sib's treatment choices are based on foundations with which you totally disagree: holistic regimens instead of 21st Century medicine, for instance, or meditation and prayer instead of radiation. These choices may make you scream and rant and throw things at the wall, but your sibling is the one who gets to make them.

This is not your illness.

What you might do in similar circumstances may be entirely different. In fact, there's an excellent chance that's the case. Actions, reactions and inactions may differ for each and every member of a large sibling cluster, but only one of you is the patient just now.

So that is where the decision making needs to ultimately land.

With the patient.

Reminder: You don't have to do everything, and you don't have to do it all right this minute.

ADDITIONAL RESOURCES

American Bar Association Commission on Law and Aging
Consumer's Tool Kit for Health Care Advance Planning
www.americanbar.org/groups/law_aging.html

Eldercare Locator
www.eldercare.gov
800.677.1116

USA.gov Senior Citizens' Resources
www.usa.gov/Topics/Seniors.shtml

• • • • •

Jessie Gruman
AfterShock: What to Do When the Doctor Gives You—or Someone You Love—a Devastating Diagnosis
Walker & Co., 2007

Michele A. Reiss
Lessons in Loss and Living: Hope and Guidance for Confronting Serious Illness and Grief
Hyperion, 2010

MEDICAL DICTIONARIES
AND REFERENCES

There are dozens of dictionaries and reference guides to symptoms. Any one will probably work just fine. Look for a fairly recent publication date on the back of the title page.

BUILDING A SIBCARE TEAM

THE PATIENT

The most important part of the entire SibCare process is the person at its center.

The patient.

You want to work with your sibling, not around him, and unless there is some legal paperwork already completed and on hand you will also *need* to work with him.

If you and other relatives are getting involved, it's likely that the patient needs more care than is currently available. But you must have your sick sibling's cooperation. Dragging a sixty-seven-year-old into the car to visit the doctor is an inauspicious beginning. And you don't even want to think about going to court to straighten matters out.

As much as possible, include the patient in decision-making large and small. You may know exactly what you would do under similar circumstances, but your sibling may have entirely different ideas.

Remember: *This is not my illness.*

YOU

If you are reading this book, you are already in deep. This is commendable. Your sibling is lucky to have you.

Take a moment for self-assessment, however, before you make commitments you can't honor. Think about the things that will make it easy for you to work with your ailing sibling. Figure out what will make matters more difficult. How much of that is you and how much is your sibling?

If you see obstacles, what is your best path to get around them?

What strengths and weaknesses do you bring to the SibCare situation? Are you working full time? Already caring for somebody else? On a limited income? Dealing with your own medical issues?

Do you live on the next block or three thousand miles away? What can you realistically offer and provide, even if everything works in your favor?

It shouldn't be too complicated to answer those questions, though it's okay to remain in denial about the answers briefly if no life-and-death decisions are immediately required. And after you've given yourself the once-over, you can cast the net a bit wider.

If you're starting from scratch, you may need to notify and recruit help from family members. This can be problematic, particularly if there has been friction of either recent or longstanding sorts between ... well, between or among any configuration of the sibs and other relatives.

If you get along with everybody involved, then you are a perfect recruiter. But be realistic. If you tend to be a little too straightforward and gruff and your sister can talk birds down out of the trees, she's the one you want making the calls for help.

From this day forward, you must also remember to take care of yourself as well as your sibling. Pamper yourself routinely and every now and then veer at least briefly into out-and-out self-indulgence.

Make some personal quiet time every day even if it means locking yourself in a closet. Take a walk around the block. Keep up on your favorite TV shows. Maintain your current pleasurable activities as much as you possibly can. Choose to be around people and places and activities that allow you to cast aside your current worries and problems.

Be sure you actually *do* these things for yourself. Slip off on personal business at regular intervals. Put it on the calendar.

I will also remind you regularly that martyrdom is a very unattractive quality.

RALLY THE TROOPS

Figure out who's available right now and work with what you've got at the beginning.

As you pull folks together, try not to be panicky. If somebody's off on a once-in-a-lifetime vacation, leave them alone for the moment. They need to be notified, of course, and perhaps pressed into service when they return, but unless it's truly a life-or-death matter, don't insist that everybody show up immediately. Staggering the timing of assistance from different people may actually help if there's a need to share responsibilities later on.

As you interact with your sib's various friends, family members, and coworkers, keep an eye out for people with useful talents or connections. Keep your options open, and try not to dump anybody into niches too quickly. Don't ignore some in-law's lawyer cousin because you're so eager to find an RN lurking in the extended family. You may need that lawyer later.

Also don't forget that enthusiasm for helping is a talent all by itself, and that simple availability can be an asset. A big one. One person who wants to help and is available can be more useful than half a dozen who think maybe they can give you a hand later. And if the enthusiasm exceeds actual usefulness, well, there's always necessary busy work to occupy the earnest incompetent.

Make notes about these people and everything else— either in your preferred digital format or on a plain, old-fashioned legal pad, and keep them accessible.

You may think you're on top of everything, but at some point you will realize that your brain has been in the Spin Dry cycle for a couple of weeks and you no longer remember anything, including all your passwords and the name of your first pet.

TYPES OF SIBCARE SITUATIONS

It can help a great deal when you're beginning to deal

with a SibCare situation to step back for a moment and determine what sort of situation it actually is. This identification will affect everything that happens from here on out. More than one of these may apply:

- Something that has already happened, carries repercussions, and will require recovery and rehabilitation. Stroke and heart attack are the two major players in this department. Serious accidents of any sort usually fit here as well.
- A scheduled event. This includes major surgery of many sorts, often the replacement of worn out body parts such as knees and hips.
- A brand new diagnosis, more or less out of the blue. Here's where everybody is likely to be in a white-hot panic, starting from scratch.
- An illness that is ongoing and likely to be progressive. Major illnesses such as diabetes, Parkinson's, Multiple Sclerosis, and Alzheimer's fall under this heading. So do a host of other diseases for which treatment may stave off advancement without an outright cure or the reclaiming of lost territory.
- Cancer. There are so many types of cancer and so many variables related to each that it really is in a category all its own.
- A mysterious malady that has yet to be diagnosed or explained. This can be the most infuriating and frustrating, because while symptoms can be addressed, it is often without certainty that the treatment is even appropriate.
- Side effects and reactions. Once you have a diagnosis and a treatment plan, an entirely different set of problems can arise from side effects and reactions related to those treatments.

COMFORT ZONES

Figure out, early on, what your own comfort zone is in

helping to care and advocate for your sibling.

In large measure, this is a matter of honest self-evaluation. You aren't doing anybody any favors if you try to take on tasks that make you uncomfortable or leave you fairly certain that you've done everything wrong.

Your sister may be sick and not tracking as well as usual, but she's known you as long as you've known her. She'll be able to tell if you are repelled by something you're trying to do for her, or if you've let yourself get hopelessly over your head. And it won't make her feel any better to realize that there's not much she can do about it.

With the understanding that you aren't looking for a new career—just trying to help somebody you care about get through a tough time—think about these questions. There are no right or wrong answers.

- Are you a nurturing caregiver, always at the ready with ice chips or a heating pad or a fluffed-up pillow?
- Will you faint if you try to change dressings or give an injection? Can you handle shunts, feeding tubes, or other unfortunate items that may have been inserted in your sibling's body? Are you able to hold a basin while somebody vomits without upchucking yourself?
- Do sick rooms in general make you claustrophobic?
- Do you deal easily with medical information and personnel?
- Does medical research thrill you, or does it give you Med Student's Syndrome, certain that you and/or your sister have every medical problem discussed on the Internet, as well as some that haven't yet reached the medical blogosphere?
- Do you keep track of appointments, pay bills promptly, and know immediately where to find whatever you may need for any given task?
- Does taking on authority figures and officious bureaucrats leave you tongue-tied and confused, or do you thrive on the sport?

- Are you gentle and deft with your hands, or do you tend to be clumsy in situations that call for precision and fine motor skills?
- Can you assemble a nourishing meal out of medically-limited ingredients and persuade somebody with no appetite to eat it?
- Are you strong enough to physically assist your ailing sibling in and out of bed, to the bathroom, and from car to wheelchair and back?
- Do you fall to pieces in the face of adversity?
- How's your poker face?
- Are you fun to be around?

Now that you've figured out your own strengths and weaknesses, ask the same questions about the others you are hoping will be part of your getting-started team. If you *are* the team, you're done. If you honestly have no idea about others, ask but make it open-ended. *Have you had much experience with sick people?* is better than *Are you going to be able to help him with the toilet?* and is likely to get the person talking in a way that will determine whether you are dealing with Florence Nightingale's latest incarnation or somebody who has fainted every single time she's had a shot.

With a little bit of luck, you'll find complementary comfort zones among the members of your caregiving team, zones that fit together into a useful whole.

YOUR SIBLINGS

If there are other siblings on the planet, you should always make an effort to include them in a SibCare crisis. Yes, even if they were headed into the Australian outback or Costa Rican jungle the last time anybody heard from them, fifteen or so years ago.

If everybody is already on pretty good terms, your sibling's bad news can be a splendid opportunity for people to rise to an occasion and share their time, talents, and resources toward the greater familial good. A noble concept, and entirely plausible for some families. This is the best of all possible worlds.

For everybody else, involving the sibs will fall somewhere on a continuum between Challenging and Downright Impossible.

Look for complementary talents. Remember that everybody can probably contribute some element, even a minor one. It may be hands-on caregiving, hospital visitation, financial management or assistance, information procurement, chauffeur service, knowing somebody with specialized relevant talents, or simply offering strong moral support.

Don't downplay moral support, either. Sometimes a sincere and heartfelt "attaboy" can bail out an otherwise awful day.

If folks are already estranged, sibling illness can lead in all sorts of different directions. It may bring everyone back together in unity, remembering all the good times, or clarify ongoing issues by recalling all the bad times. Parents add more spice to any of these stews, and they don't even have to be alive to do it.

It's also not uncommon for at least one person to be seriously on the outs with somebody else. In some families, flowcharts are required to chronicle ongoing feuds.

Serious illness can whomp the hell out of any relationship, even a really good one. If you're starting off in the hole vis-à-vis camaraderie, it's probably a good idea to look for common ground and proceed with extreme caution. "How about those Yankees!?"

It might not work.

But attempting to include the other siblings is almost always worth a shot. There may be some detached way even the most seriously estranged sibling can help. And keep in mind that the Internet makes it wonderfully easy to interact both en masse and at a distance. Texting is also a useful way to exchange specific information without having somebody difficult in your face or shouting in your ear.

If a sibling absolutely refuses to help, let it go and move on. You may get some assistance from that sib later. Or not. Either way, you need to save your energy for other battles.

CHALLENGES OF A SIBLING TEAM

Is it better to have more siblings, or less?

This is a question you probably thought about a lot when you were a kid. You wanted more or less, different genders, older, or younger. Maybe like Goldilocks, you found the existing family configuration just right. But don't pretend sibling demographics never crossed your mind.

If there are several of you, SibCare can be much less burdensome, but remember you are dealing with personalities and behavior patterns that are well established. This can cut either way. It may mean that a finely-tuned, precision team is falling into place and will work together flawlessly. It can also mean chaos, with or without an overlay of organization.

Somebody needs to be in charge and coordinate, however loosely. The more people involved on essentially the same level of participation, the greater the likelihood of confusion or duplication of efforts. You also need a little flexibility to allow for buck-passing and flaking out. Folks scattered hither and yon in different time zones can be a complication, too.

You may uncover other hidden problems, as well.

Did one of your other siblings die young? If so, the current illness is bound to bring up all kinds of issues for everybody. Some things we just didn't know how to talk about before. If you lost a brother or sister as a child—whether to illness, accident, or cruel turn of fate—there are likely to be lingering questions and issues. It's entirely possible that you've never talked about it at all. With mortality punching you once again in the eye, it may be time to start talking about what happened, with the others who were also there.

Just try to keep it out of the way of the primary issue: your living sibling's current SibCare situation.

PARENTS

If you have living parents, they will automatically be a part of the equation, whether as useful and active participants, obstacles to be circumvented, or somewhere in between.

Parents in good health and of sound mind are useful in many situations, particularly if folks all get along and the sick person is young, with or without children. But as parental age climbs, you may find that the parental unit(s) are more trouble than help.

For one thing, they are likely to have a laundry list of their own physical problems and issues, not to mention any caregiving you might already be extending in that direction. Parents can also be bossy, even when they are weak, and habits are so deeply ingrained that people fall right into behavioral patterns. Memory issues are a real concern here, too.

Plus, there are few sights less appealing than a ninety-two-year-old drama queen who thinks she's being upstaged by one of her children.

If older parents are around, you're likely to hear a lot of: "Why couldn't it have been me? I've had a good life." This sentiment crosses many cultural lines. And if parents are impaired themselves, you may find it easier to not share all information about your sibling's problems, particularly if there isn't a lot of information at the moment.

Remember when you were a teenager and you stopped telling your parents everything? It may be time to take up that habit again, for everybody's peace of mind.

YOUR SIBLING'S SPOUSAL UNIT(S)

There's no simple answer to the question of how the people that your sibling has married will fit into the overall SibCare picture.

Of course, if a current spouse is actively involved right now, you are far less likely to be orchestrating anything. There's a pecking order here. Medical personnel, bureaucrats, and anybody else involved will automatically look first to the husband or wife, then to children. Only if these all come up empty is a sibling likely to be considered.

But matters are often messier than that, even if the marriage is intact. Even if the marriage is *fantastic*, regularly cited by everybody in your sister's universe as perfect. Being a good caregiver or advocate calls for a different skill set than being a good spouse, though overlap certainly exists. If your sister's husband communicates poorly or your brother's wife falls to pieces, your help may be needed just to keep matters on track.

Sibling divorces in the landscape offer a lot of attendant baggage that you probably tried to avoid while those divorces were actually in process. Nobody is obligated to involve a spouse from a marriage that ended bitterly, though if shared children are part of the package, that isn't really optional.

Indeed, former spouses may want to be involved, and may have important skills and connections that can help everybody. If that's the case, roll with it so long as your sibling doesn't balk. And if the sib balks and the help is important, see what you can manage on the QT. (Without forgetting, of course, that this is not your illness.)

Actual marriage is not required, either.

The mother of the two de facto stepkids who cared for my brother in his final three years was never married to him, though they had lived together for six years, a quarter-century earlier. She wisely advised her children at the outset not to take on responsibility for him, though luckily for the Cannon family they didn't listen. And while she never assumed primary caregiving, her presence and attention was an enormous help to my sister and me, since she was some 1800 miles closer to our brother than we were. She also knew everybody in the area where he was now living, since she'd grown up there and was now a sergeant on the local police force. (I would never have imagined myself saying this forty years ago, but I love being tight with the cops.)

Sometimes, as Willie Nelson wrote, "Miracles appear in the strangest of places."

Case in point are those two amazing young people who watched out for my brother, under the equally watchful eye of the ex he never married. The Cannon family is here to tell you that anything can happen.

KIDS AND STEPKIDS

Your sibling's children and stepchildren come first, though your own kids and other nieces and nephews may also be helpful.

To figure out how your nieces and nephews will fit into the larger scheme of things, start with some basics.

How old are they? Are they working? In school? Married? Where do the grown children live? Do they have their own children, and what kind of relationship do *those* kids have with the grandparent in question?

And perhaps most important, how do they get along with the ailing parent? Who'll be a help and who'll be a hindrance? Everybody's carrying baggage and if anything needs to be aired, it's nice to find out early on.

Remember each new generation has their *own* sibling clusters and relationships, not to mention their own versions of sibling issues. It's a never-ending cycle. Keep in mind also that you'll also get very different responses and help from a 23-year-old than a 43-year-old, though in either case temperament always trumps age.

Very young children are an entirely different and much more complicated matter. Here the issues are both philosophical—*What should they be told?*—and practical—*Who's keeping an eye on them?* A particularly tough scenario is the under-eighteen child whose parents fought an ugly divorce.

If there have been divorces, the landscape is strewn with additional land mines. Ugly or bitter divorces leave scars that aren't always obvious to anyone until times of crisis. If your nephew sided with Mom and now Dad is suddenly very ill, there's a world of opportunity for guilt and self-recrimination. We can only hope that Mom isn't still saying, "I wish he were dead."

Multiple divorces increase the likelihood of personnel problems exponentially.

OTHER FAMILY MEMBERS

Here's where you may just get really lucky, depending on how you define "family." Don't be too picky about that definition, either, because the most helpful family members may turn out to be people you barely even thought of in the first place.

This is a catch-all category for cousins, in-laws, in-laws of in-laws, exes, and spin-offs in every possible direction. Remember that guy whose sister used to be married to your cousin? Wasn't he an accountant? Even if you aren't actively recruiting this kind of backup staff, keep likely helpers in the back of your mind as you run across them.

And since your mind probably isn't lending itself to that kind of filing right now, write it down in a notebook, or make an electronic note in a place where you'll be able to find it later.

CASTING THE NET WIDER

You might discover that you are still extremely short-handed after you have exhausted all family members who might be able to help. You may, in fact, be all there is.

Don't panic yet.

Your sister hasn't been living in a vacuum all this time. Odds are good that she has some friends. Start there. Are there old friends you've heard her talk about, maybe kids you all knew growing up together? College classmates, or buddies from military service, or the Peace Corps?

If these friendships remain current and local, find these folks and talk to them. They may have already found you, or surfaced at the hospital, or even been the one who called you in the first place. Ask questions, particularly if you know they are close to your sibling and may be aware of things that family members are not.

If you can't come up with any obvious friends, step back and think about how your sibling likes to spend her spare time. Most people have a couple of significant activities or organizations in their lives. The key is to crack one or more of these groups. Ideally this will produce a helpful soul who can direct you to people in that group most likely to have information you need or be inclined to help.

Possibilities to consider:
- *Work.* This is true even if your sibling is officially retired, and it may go beyond current coworkers. Don't forget unions and business associations, or previous jobs which may have led to continuing friendships.
- *Church.* If your sibling is actively involved in a faith community of almost any kind, this is likely to be a treasure trove of caring and concerned people, some of whom will want to help and are likely to show up when they say they will. Many religious communities have internal groups or procedures for helping one another in times of need. Their beliefs may differ from yours, but help is help.
- *Neighbors.* Ring a few doorbells and introduce yourself. Your sib may have some friends in the neighborhood, but they won't necessarily live next door, since this is not a TV sitcom. However, the people next door may have noticed that your brother always goes over and talks to the guy who lives on the corner, or know that your sister and the woman in the red brick house down the block raised their kids together. If you stumble upon the neighborhood busybody, you may not get entirely accurate information, but you're sure to come away with an earful. Somewhere in there may be exactly the nugget you need.
- *Military buddies.* If your sibling hangs out at the VFW or American Legion, check it out.
- *Fitness and sports friends.* If your sibling is involved in some kind of regular sports activity, even if it's just watching football with the gang, this is a potential gold

mine. If actual sports participation or a health club is involved, you have the added advantage of people who may be in pretty solid physical condition. This also includes things like yoga and Pilates and exercise classes of all sorts. Also hunting and fishing buddies.

- *Book clubs, craft connections, organizational memberships.* This may be five former coworkers who get together monthly with some wine and a book they've all supposedly read, or the folks in a quilting circle, or AAUW, or Rotary, or Kiwanis, or the Masonic Lodge.
- *Fellow volunteers.* Your sib may be involved in some kind of volunteer organization, which by definition means people who are interested in being useful and helpful. Bingo!

YOUR OWN SUPPORT SYSTEM

It's easy to forget this one, which is terrifically important.

While you're involved with your sibling, you are under a lot of stress. And you probably weren't floating in a cloud of butterflies when all this started. Perhaps you were already under significant stress from other directions when your world suddenly changed its parameters.

One way to take care of yourself through all this is to identify your own support system, and to learn how to lean on those folks when you need to.

You may have old friends from when you started kindergarten, or from when your kids started kindergarten. You might have a BFF you just met last year. You've also got neighbors, coworkers from various jobs, and maybe members and leaders from your own church or faith community. Maybe you're tight with the women in your exercise class, or the people in your book club, or your tennis regulars. Don't forget the guys you go fishing with up north every summer. Or the girlfriends who gather every winter for a long weekend in Vegas.

One thing may surprise you as you expand the circle of

those aware of your ongoing family situation. Other folks you know may be in similar or related situations. They're even more likely to know somebody in their own circle who's going through a variant of what you are. There's a lot of SibCare going around. You just don't realize it because sick siblings don't always come up right away when you run into people at the grocery store or gym.

So keep an eye and ear out for others with SibCare responsibilities or stories among your friends, coworkers, and acquaintances. You can form special alliances with those folks, and learn from each other, since each of you understands the situation and gets it.

And speaking of *getting it,* prepare yourself for the reality that a lot of people don't, or won't, or can't. One excellent way to do that is to read the stories of people who have faced the same challenges you're looking at right now.

• • • • •

PEOPLE WHO HAVE BEEN THERE

Elisa Albert, ed.
Freud's Blind Spot: 23 Original Essays on Cherished, Estranged, Lost, Hurtful, Hopeful, Complicated Siblings
Free Press, 2010

Nell Casey, ed.
An Uncertain Inheritance: Writers on Caring for Family
William Morrow, 2007

Richard M. Cohen
Strong at the Broken Places: Voices of Illness, a Chorus of Hope
HarperCollins, 2008

The Healing Project
Voices of Caregiving
LaChance Publishing, 2009

Don Meyer, ed.
Thicker Than Water: Essays by Adult Siblings of People with Disabilities
Woodbine House, 2009

Randy Pausch with Jeffrey Zaslow
The Last Lecture
Hyperion, 2008

Julie K. Silver, ed.
What Helped Get Me Through: Cancer Survivors Share Wisdom and Hope
American Cancer Society, 2009

Lisa Snyder
Speaking Our Minds: Personal Reflections from Individuals with Alzheimer's
W.H. Freeman & Co., 1999

Victoria Zackheim, ed.
Exit Laughing: How Humor Takes the Sting Out of Death
North Atlantic Books, 2012

INFORMATION GATHERING

AND ADVOCACY

Various stages of your particular SibCare situation will require different types of information. A lot of this is simple common sense.

If you're in the middle of a crisis, your concerns will be different than if you're making adjustments in the aftermath of that crisis. Faced with an unfamiliar diagnosis, you may feel urgency about medical research. If your sibling's living space must be adapted for new mobility issues, you'll want to explore accessibility and modification possibilities. When the treatment becomes more onerous than the affliction, you'll be looking for palliatives and relief. And a desk overflowing with unpaid bills requires a different skill set altogether.

IS THIS TRULY A SURPRISE?

If the medical issue is a longstanding problem—for example, deteriorating joints that started back with high school basketball—there's not much to report. If it's a chronic condition that's been around for a while but is suddenly kicking up a fuss, you've probably already got some groundwork in.

It may also be something that you already know way too much about and were hoping was gone for good—now making an unwelcome return appearance. You may not need to do much medical research in a case like this, but you will certainly need to allow some time for sorrow and denial. If you've been down this road more than once, it's even easier to feel crushed by disappointment at having to face down the enemy one more time.

Indulge yourself in grief for a while.

I noticed at various stages of my brother's illness I had to start all over again with Elisabeth Kubler-Ross's five stages of grief: Denial, Anger, Bargaining, Depression, Acceptance. Yes, these are supposed to be only associated with death, and they certainly fit there. But serious illness is a form of psychic death and emotional trauma, and they fit pretty neatly there as well.

I also noticed that I ran through them faster each time, often not even bothering to stop at Bargaining and Depression.

WHAT FRESH HELL IS THIS?

Brand new organic medical complaints can get a lot trickier, especially those occurring in people who've previously been very healthy or who are major league hypochondriacs.

In the first case, it's often because the previously healthy go into denial and assume they can fix the problem with more exercise or better diet. Steve Jobs is the classic example of this syndrome, and he paid dearly for it. As for hypochondriacs, they're the Boy Who Cried Wolf and it may be a while before anyone takes their complaints seriously, including their primary care physicians.

Most people fall somewhere in the middle, however.

ACCIDENTS, AUTO AND OTHERWISE

Even something as straightforward as an auto accident where another driver ran into your sibling's car may have a hidden subtext.

The key question here is: "What was happening immediately before the accident?" Did your brother black out for a moment, or did his foot jerk on the pedal, or was he too distracted to notice that the light had changed?

If there's an accident report, it can be useful to see it. Also necessary, in case the report seems to be about an occurrence very different from what your sibling has recounted. By simple virtue of being an Official Document, a police report carries more weight than accounts from witnesses and/or participants, both legally and with insurance companies. This can come back to bite you, so check it out now.

This is particularly true if others were hurt and/or your sibling was the party at fault.

Even non-injury auto accidents often have legal repercussions which need to be addressed. If it's messy and your sibling isn't in great shape, getting power of attorney to handle this specific situation on your brother's behalf may be necessary. And if it's *really* messy, he probably needs legal representation, either through his own insurance company or independently or both.

Where any accidents are concerned, you should try to conduct separate sibling conversations about medical and legal problems, two entirely different sets of issues. Since you're going to have to deal with the medical problems regardless of what happens on the legal side, it makes sense to start with the medical.

BECOME AN ADVOCATE, OR FIND ONE

When you most need to stand up for your rights and ask intelligent questions and process the responses thoughtfully to make good decisions is too often the time when you are least able to.

When you're sick. Really, really sick.

What you need most of all just then is an advocate.

A flat out, take-no-prisoners advocate who combines the genial charm of a golden retriever with the wiliness of a feral cat and the tenacity of a terrier. Somebody to take on the medical personnel and hold off anybody who's giving you a hard time for other reasons and keep the affairs of your life running as smoothly as possible under the circumstances. Somebody capable of doing whatever needs to be done to promote your greater good.

It sounds like a *Help Wanted* ad for Wonder Woman or Superman, but don't despair or sell yourself short. You might be a lot better at this than you think.

For one thing, it's often easier to speak up and stand up for somebody else than to do the same for yourself. In this case there's no question in your mind that you're advocating for a very worthy cause, whether it's to take care of your sister for the duration or get yourself extricated as quickly as possible.

There are several excellent resources for information on advocacy, complete with checklists and forms you can follow. Many advocacy books grew out of somebody's personal experience and all are rich with personal detail.

Not everybody is cut out to be an advocate, and there's no dishonor if you just aren't right for that position. Your sibling can still use the service, however. Make a particular effort to recruit other family members or perhaps one of your sibling's friends to take on advocacy.

Advocacy can also be split up. One person might be great with the medical stuff but lousy at charming creditors, while somebody else faints at blood despite razor-sharp business communication skills.

Cobble together whoever you have and the talents represented and give it your best shot.

You'll be better at it than you think. Trust me.

GETTING INFORMATION OUT OF THE MEDICAL STOCKADE

It used to be a lot easier to get medical information from health care professionals. Indeed, in olden times some of these folks were incredible blabbermouths. Oliver Wendell Holmes, Sr., was Nathaniel Hawthorne's personal physician, and he actually published an article about his patient's health concerns in *The Atlantic Monthly* after Hawthorne died.

The information-sharing bar has been raised considerably since then.

In our own lifetimes, everything was supposed to be confidential and for the most part it was. Of course if your doctor's receptionist was a busybody and a gossip, you and your privacy were screwed.

The biggest change has been on a more bureaucratic

and Big Brother level. Suddenly everybody's personal medical business was built into all kinds of databases, essentially available to any fourteen-year-old hacker with a desire for information on Elmer Larson's chilblains. Then insurance companies began using this giant slush-fund of electronic data to deny or cancel coverage (sometimes in the middle of chemotherapy) to patients who had neglected to mention a childhood infected hangnail on their applications. Insurance employees got awards and bonuses for cancelling the largest number of policies.

So things tightened up.

The Health Insurance Portability and Accountability Act of 1996 (HIPAA) made it far more difficult for your private information to be shared, even with your own close relatives and loved ones. (Insurance company databases, alas, appear to be forever and beyond anyone's reach or control, though they are less frightening now that nobody can be denied health insurance for pre-existing conditions.) HIPAA privacy is a dandy idea in general, but it can be a real pain and problem if your loved one is in the Emergency Room or ICU and nobody is sharing information with you because the paperwork is not in order.

To be sure that you can receive medical information from any person or group or institution involved in the care of your sibling, that sibling should sign a HIPAA form giving that authorization. HIPAA forms are available in any medical office and can be rescinded at any time. Once that paperwork is in place, medical people can speak freely with you.

Failure to sign a HIPAA form does not, however, automatically preclude the sharing of information unless the patient specifically objects. This is particularly true in emergency situations or when the patient is incapacitated. Nor does it prevent anyone from *sharing* medical information with the patient's medical team.

Verbal authorization can be used as well, though a signature is always better.

VISITING THE DOCTOR

If you're accompanying your sister to a medical appointment, get ready in advance. Don't try to wing it. Make lists and write out questions. Use a tablet, or a dedicated little notebook, or go all out and carry a legal pad. Leave space to jot down answers and don't forget to bring your own pen. Two pens, in case one of them runs out of ink. Get questions and concerns from your ailing sibling well in advance. If you give her a chance to think about it for a day or two, she's likely to remember something that might otherwise be overlooked.

Practice asking questions in the mirror if you're nervous.

If the doctor or practitioner you're seeing raises new topics or issues, follow up on those before starting on your list, and take notes. If your sibling is in the room while you're asking questions, pay attention to her. And let her speak for herself if she's willing and able.

Sick people *hate* being ignored or talked about as if they aren't even in the room. Nobody is pleased to be treated that way, of course, but it happens a lot more often with sick people.

Remember that there's a fine line between speaking on somebody's behalf and taking over. Try to know where that line is, particularly when you're crossing it.

It is generally wise to accompany your sibling into the examining room, but discuss this in advance so it doesn't feel like an ambush or set off a scene in the waiting room. And for heaven's sake, respect your sibling's privacy if something potentially embarrassing is scheduled. You don't need to be in the room for the pelvic or prostate exam.

Your sibling probably doesn't want to be there, either.

Be very polite and listen carefully.

Ask questions if you don't understand something and repeat after me: **There are no stupid questions.** If you aren't getting the information you want, rephrase your question. Dumb it down or crank it up a notch, whichever seems appropriate.

Keep in mind as well that while you may not need all this information just now, at some future point you may want it desperately. So write everything down and keep those notes in a safe, accessible spot. If they're digital, back them up.

Look for specific answers where it's possible, but don't be surprised or disheartened if there aren't many for a while. Often in a medical crisis, it simply isn't possible to tell what is going to happen—until it happens. When you're in a medical waiting game, every minute seems an eternity. Then—*Blam!*—decisions must be made. ASAP.

It's dreadful on everybody, but that's the way it is. Your armor in this battle is whatever knowledge you are able to accumulate along the way.

Ingratiate yourself with the doctor's office staff. The doc may ultimately call the shots, but it's the receptionists and nurses and techs and office assistants you'll deal with most. Keep in mind that these are people who voluntarily went into helping professions, and assume that all of you want the very best outcomes for your sibling.

Always, always, always be polite and gracious on the phone. Yelling at the office gatekeeper isn't going to get your brother better treatment and it could land you on hold for twenty minutes. Repeatedly.

Don't say something is an emergency if it isn't. In a genuine emergency, you should be calling 911 anyway. If you have to leave a voice mail message, be concise and accurate and avoid melodrama. Repeat your name, your sibling's name, and your phone number at the end of the message.

Pay attention to names and try to remember them. Smile at everybody, even if it's through your tears. If you visit a particular office regularity, it doesn't hurt to occasionally bring flowers or goodies. This needn't be designer chocolates or long-stemmed roses. A box of Girl Scout cookies or a cute little plant from the grocery store will work just fine.

DO YOUR RESEARCH

Most topics discussed in this book have a list of specific resources for obtaining additional information. If you're in a hurry, you can download many of the books onto your Kindle or other e-reader and get started while your cup of tea is steeping. Or you can wait till morning and call the 800 number of a disease foundation and talk to a real person who can provide you with more specific resources and local contact information.

The key here is taking that first step. You may be (justifiably) afraid of what you're going to learn, but you may also discover that you're worrying needlessly about something that actually isn't important. Remember those motivators that Social Studies teachers used to put around their classrooms?

Knowledge is power.

SEEK ASSISTANCE
WHEN YOU NEED IT

If you aren't the best person to tackle a particular problem or challenge, try to find somebody who is, and pay that person if necessary. Delegating or hiring out a chore may mean that something won't be done perfectly, i.e. to your own exacting specifications, but this is a bullet you sometimes need to bite.

Illness is just another manifestation of an imperfect world. You are not responsible for either the state of the world or the current health of your sibling.

You can't do everything, know everything, and be everything—and you shouldn't try. This is particularly true if you're normally an overachiever, a worrywart, or both.

On a more practical note, if you try to do everything yourself and do it perfectly, you'll wear yourself down to a nub. Or you'll start complaining, because it's just all too much (which it is). Whining will discourage folks from leaping forward to assist.

Help is what you really want, isn't it? So make at least a token effort at being the kind of person people want to assist.

Martyrdom is not just an unattractive quality. It's also lonely.

THAT #*$&# PAPERWORK

Various paperwork chores demand attention at the outset of any SibCare situation. Just about everybody hates this, both because it deals with uncomfortable issues and because it's, well, *paperwork.*

So get over it. We're all grownups now, and the chapters on "The Paperwork Morass" and "Legal Paperwork" will help you through it all. For the moment, start with a basic checklist:

- What kind of insurance does your sibling have: health, long-term care, cancer, accident, disability?
- Does any proposed treatment require special insurance company approval that has to get started right this second?
- Does your sibling qualify for fast-tracked Social Security Disability through the Compassionate Allowances Program? A list of over a hundred very serious diagnoses moves you to the head of the SSD line. Not a list you'd ever choose to be on, but useful if you need more help in a hurry. www.ssa.gov/compassionateallowances.
- Does your sibling have advance directives for health care?
- Has your sibling designated somebody to have financial power of attorney?
- Does your sibling have an established will or trust?
- Is there a whole life insurance policy with an end-of-life waiver allowing your sibling to draw on the policy for nursing home or hospice care? If that isn't already in effect, can you add it now?

TECHNOLOGY

Make technology work for you as you get things set up. We live in a marvelous age, when digital media and electronics are changing at dizzying rates. Even better, other people have done a lot of the groundwork for you, sometimes for free.

This includes websites with ready-to-go templates for legal documents and to coordinate care and information with however wide a circle you choose. You can regulate access to these sites and make them as private as you want them to be, and as detailed as you need them to be. There's more on this in the chapters on "Legal Paperwork" and "Caregiving."

Pay attention to who you're working with, however. If you camp out in the Apple line on every release day, you undoubtedly lead a rich and fulfilled technological life. But if everybody else is back somewhere in the Princess phone era, dumb down your technological communication plans so that the others can participate, even if it means going to such anachronistic systems as wall calendars, notebooks, and the US Pony Express.

You may devise a brilliant, multi-device technical communication system that can be synched to your own private family website as well as for eighteen different people in eleven different locations.

But it's a Pyrrhic victory if seventeen of them have no clue how to use or access that system.

THE BIG PICTURE

Try to keep at least partial focus on the Big Picture.
This can vary greatly.

One sibling may be about to replace a hip that's been problematic since that motorcycle crash, with the promise of greater mobility and renewed energy, maybe even a return to rock climbing. Another faces treatment for a Glioblastoma that will likely claim her within a year.

You are never required to entirely abandon hope. Scientists work tirelessly in labs around the globe on medical research, and one of them may be about to announce a breakthrough that will change everything for your sibling.

It can happen.

It *does* happen, though not nearly often enough.

It may be that you find the Big Picture just too tough to look at immediately, or even for a while. Tiptoe around it, then, and deal with the small, manageable decisions of the moment.

I spent a lot of time ignoring things related to my brother's medical, personal, and financial woes because, after all, the world might blow up tomorrow. This didn't change anything, but it did let me get to tomorrow again and again and again.

What's more, some of the things that I ignored went away on their own or resolved themselves peacefully, occasionally in my brother's favor.

Procrastination can sometimes be its own reward.

LIFE IS A TWELVE-STEP PROGRAM

Odds are excellent that you know people who are committed to various Twelve-Step recovery programs. You may be in one yourself. One reason why these programs work is that they rest on a simple premise: One Day at a Time.

One Day at a Time is a concept that has helped a lot of people deal with problems that seemed previously insurmountable. Try to apply the same principle to your family's SibCare crisis. Continue the same pattern when it downgrades to a SibCare situation.

There will be periods when it is all you can do to put one foot in front of the other. Those are times when it is useful to think of your current life as being one hour at a time.

You don't have to solve all the problems at once. You don't even need to *address* all the problems at once. If some of these problems happen to be your other siblings—and trust me, this happens all the time—you may be able to head off a looming confrontation by focusing on the immediate future. After all, you just have to get along for today.

ADVOCACY RESOURCES

Patient Advocate Foundation
www.patientadvocate.org
800.532.5274

PULSE Patient Safety and Advocacy
www.pulseamerica.org

• • • • •

Jari Holland Buck
Hospital Stay Handbook: A Guide to Becoming a Patient Advocate for Your Loved Ones
Llewellyn Publications, 2007

Elizabeth S. Cohen
The Empowered Patient: How to Get the Right Diagnosis, Buy the Cheapest Drugs, Beat Your Insurance Company, and Get the Best Medical Care Every Time
Ballantine, 2010

Ellen Menard
The Not So Patient Advocate: How to Get the Health Care You Need Without Fear or Frustration
Bardolf & Company, 2009

Brian and Gerri Monaghan
The Power of Two: Surviving Serious Illness with an Attitude and an Advocate
Workman, 2009

Andrew Schorr
The Web-Savvy Patient: An Insider's Guide to Navigating the Internet When Facing Medical Crisis
CreateSpace, 2011

Trisha Torrey
The Health Advocate's Start and Grow Your Own Practice Handbook: A Step by Step Guide
DiagKNOWsis Media, 2012

James Thomas Williams
The Patient Advocate's Handbook: 300 Questions and Answers to Help You Care for Your Loved One at the Hospital and at Home
Panglossian Press, 2010

LEARNING WHAT YOU NEED TO KNOW

WHAT *DO* YOU ACTUALLY NEED TO KNOW?

Trying to figure out how to obtain VA benefits for a reluctant Vietnam vet? Grappling with rigid dietary restrictions for somebody who has always eaten whatever she pleases? Wondering how you can get a wheelchair down that narrow corridor, never mind up the stairs? Looking for information about a disease you have never heard of before?

A world of information is out there to help, starting with the good old-fashioned printed word. Innumerable websites are devoted to different diseases, or to straightening out credit problems, or to caregiving at a distance. It's almost impossible to find a problem that somebody on the Internet doesn't claim to have a solution for.

Sometimes there is an embarrassment of riches.

Certain well-funded foundations for diseases with large numbers of affected patients—cancer and diabetes spring immediately to mind—offer so many official publications that it's hard to even know where to start. And that's before you begin to sift through official government publications, and books by doctors with special treatment regimens, and personal accounts from celebrities and plain folks who have either conquered an affliction or learned to live with it.

In the bibliographies and additional resources scattered throughout this book, I've included lists of recent titles for many subjects. For the most part these are ten years old or less—generally much less, since medical information changes rapidly in the 21st Century.

I pass these references along with the understanding that I am merely a conduit.

I can't vouch for any of it. I am not a medical doctor. I have never even played one on television.

I did the research to show the range of what is available, but you are on your own to follow up and decide whether an information source is worthy of your time and attention.

I wish somebody had done the same for me, frankly, so that when I needed to learn about brain tumors or strokes or seizures or lymphoma in a hurry, I would at least have had some clue how to start. Since I generally thrive on research, this suggests to me that perhaps everybody is paralyzed for a while when up against a new medical obstacle.

In cases where I've found a resource or a book particularly helpful, I'll mention it specifically and tell you why.

In assembling these references, I've tried to be comprehensive.

This means I wasn't always able to be terribly picky. If there's only one book on your sister's disease and it's by a doctor you've never heard of, you're still going to want that book even though it's poorly written and looks like it was typeset by second graders. On the other hand, there are hundreds of personal accounts by breast cancer survivors.

I always include subtitles, even when they are longer than the first chapter. If you can eliminate or include something on your "Check this out" list based on a subtitle, then everybody gains some time.

Some diseases just aren't common enough to have their own websites, or books about them, not to mention treatments and ongoing medical research. Commonly known as "orphan diseases" and often the subject of heartbreaking Lifetime channel movies, these afflictions are tough to diagnose. Once you have a diagnosis, you will probably have to learn more through very specific online searches, and you may even be lucky enough to find an online support group with relatives of four of the eleven other patients in the country.

CELEBRITY DISEASES

As harsh as it sounds, the best thing that can happen to someone with a disease is for a celebrity to contract it.

If the celebrity is beloved, all the better, and there is no more appropriate illustration than former Mouseketeer Annette Funicello. When Annette was first diagnosed with Multiple Sclerosis, she kept it private, but after a period of time (and some slimy tabloid coverage suggesting that publicly-observed balance problems were alcohol-related), she did go public.

And my, oh my, did people ever start to discuss MS when she did that! If everybody's favorite Mouseketeer could end up in a wheelchair with an incurable and progressive disease, it could obviously happen to anybody. Annette formed a foundation, though there were already several Multiple Sclerosis foundations in existence. All of them got more attention and greater donations because of her misfortune.

What Annette did for MS, Michael J. Fox has done for Parkinson's Disease, Patrick Swayze did for pancreatic cancer, and Jay Monahan did for colon cancer. Monahan's celebrity actually came secondhand through his widow, Katie Couric, who kept attention on colon cancer to the extent of undergoing on-the-air colonoscopies. The list of famous women with breast cancer would run for pages, though much credit goes to Betty Ford for bringing mastectomies out of the medical closet (as well as for making it okay for upper-middle-class women to admit to addiction problems).

Ted Kennedy brought attention to brain tumors and Glen Campbell to Alzheimer's and it's safe to say that both of them would rather have not become the poster boys for those diseases.

The good news is that each time a celebrity gets a rotten diagnosis and goes public, there's an uptick in folks who go in for a checkup, or schedule that overdue colonoscopy, or sneak a peek at the list of troubling behaviors signaling the possible onset of Alzheimer's. Talk shows featuring what used to be called "women's issues" discuss the disease du jour and may even showcase the patient of honor.

Research donations jump and benefits are performed. Foundations are established, usually bearing the celebrity's name, though even this sad form of fame can be fleeting. The former Yul Brynner Head and Neck Cancer Foundation is now known simply as the Head and Neck Cancer Alliance. *Da svidanya, Taras Bulba.*

"LET YOUR FINGERS DO THE WALKING"

Sometimes the easy and obvious route is also the best.

If you don't feel up to wading through lists of books, or venturing into unfamiliar areas of the Internet, or even taking a brief drive to the local library, you can probably manage a phone call.

Most major diseases have a foundation or two of their own, and more obscure medical problems are generally subsumed under related ones. You can learn about Peripheral Artery Disease through the American Heart Association, for instance.

So start with the most promising sounding foundation, which may even be one that you've heard of or donated to. Look for a toll-free number and give them a call. Tell them you're a family member of somebody who's just been diagnosed and that you would like information about that disease, any local resources they're aware of, and copies of any relevant free literature.

The people who answer these toll-free lines are usually helpful, informed, and compassionate. They may have personal experience with the disease. They understand that you have just been hit by a freight train and will try to answer your questions and acquaint you with other appropriate information sources. They may be able to steer you in a direction you hadn't even considered, or to alert you to a support group in your own or a nearby community.

If you are fortunate enough to be given a local contact, follow up on it promptly. When people say they want to help others through these organizations, they mean it. And there's nobody as useful or comforting as somebody who has been traveling on the same path you're just starting down.

Even when it's a particularly wretched path.

A WORD OF CAUTION

As Abraham Lincoln once noted, not everything on the Internet is true. Keep your BS Detector set to *High* as you conduct Internet research.

Repeat after me: **If it sounds too good to be true, it probably is.**

THE LIBRARY RULES

Remember the public library?

When I was a kid, my family used to walk once a week down to the firehouse where the Chicago Public Library Bookmobile parked on Mondays. There weren't very many books in that Bookmobile, but every week I found something of interest. I worked my way through all of the books about girls who went to New York City and had Interesting Careers, books with titles like *Susan Perry, Illustrator.* I read all the nurse books, of course, expecting to go into the family trade of medicine, though I'm darned if I recall a single volume with a title along the lines of *Taffy Cannon, Doctor.*

Every now and then we would go instead to the Walker Branch Library, a trip necessitating a ride in my mother's '54 Chevy station wagon, Mary Jane. The Walker Branch was (and is) a venerable brick building with larger collections of everything than the Bookmobile offered. Here I began checking out adult mysteries by Charlotte Armstrong and Agatha Christie, and here I researched term papers on the history of the dictionary and literary censorship as a high school student. What a bookish nerd I was!

Your library experiences may be very different, but here's the key connection: Most of us had them. Whether it was the school library or the county library or the church library or the bookmobile or just the neighbor across the street with extensive woodworking texts (or, in my case, every Perry Mason that Erle Stanley Gardner ever dictated) it was a critical part of our development.

Guess what? The library is still a pretty great place, even in this world of seventy-inch television screens and warp-speed Internet.

Most importantly, it usually features a reference librarian who can help you find what you need.

Trust me on this one: The reference librarian is your friend. These people purely love to do research, to hunt down that elusive fact or help figure out precisely what book you saw in Milwaukee last year, the one about finance with the green cover. They know the Dewey Decimal System inside out and how certain subjects are oddly categorized so that you might miss them. Sometimes they can lead you right to the shelf and the book with the information you need.

In many libraries, they can also help you manage Internet research, sometimes on library computers or tablets. A growing number of libraries now also offer free Wi-Fi, allowing patrons to use their own laptops, tablets, and phones.

SUPPORT GROUPS

There are three different types of support group situations: in-person, online, and shared caregiving, which is actually a hybrid of the first two. The sooner you look for them, the better.

Healthfinder.gov is a good jumping off point for all manner of support group information, online and otherwise. When you connect with the Wellington's Wallop Foundation, you can ask them for leads or prowl around their website for links. You can also plug "support groups for Wellington's Wallop" into a search engine and see what comes up.

IN-PERSON SUPPORT GROUPS

The in-person support group is what we've all seen on

TV and in movies, where everybody sits on folding chairs, drinks bad coffee, and shares their concerns and suggestions. The benefits of such groups are plentiful, starting with the basic reality that these other people are *right there*. You don't have to call them up or email them or try to find them on a disease website that defies all navigation logic.

They can offer you a hug, pass you a Kleenex, meet you for breakfast, and maybe even come up with a brilliant local solution to a very specific problem.

Hospitals often provide space for such groups and may facilitate them as well. Disease foundations may either sponsor them from afar or provide links to what's available in your area. Alzheimer's (and other) support groups are sometimes available through senior centers or retirement communities.

If you find one that is suited to you and your situation, you've struck gold.

In-person support groups may also prove inadequate or inappropriate for your particular needs. If the folks in the available support group are grieving the recent loss of loved ones and you're in full disease-fighting mode, this may not be the place for you.

Check out anything that sounds promising, but don't feel obligated to stick around if you aren't connecting with the others or benefitting from what's going on there.

ONLINE SUPPORT GROUPS

Online support groups can also be lifesavers, occasionally literally.

I've participated in a number of these over the years, both as research for writing projects and because somebody I cared about had a particular illness or problem.

Such groups may be the best source available for honest, helpful information. These are people who are either down in the trenches with you right now, or who have weathered the situation long enough to be able to sort out what's necessary, what's helpful, and what's ridiculous.

Listservs are available through Groups.Yahoo.com,

Groups.Google.com, and also through various disease and government websites.

Here's how these groups generally work: Members send posts to a central email address, which then distributes them to the other members, whether there are fourteen or fourteen hundred. Members may respond to the entire group (most common) or directly to the original poster asking for information or help. Other groups create threads dealing with specific issues and you can join the ones that are relevant to you.

You may need to join several lists before you find one that works for you.

Look for lists that have large numbers of members, have been around for a few years or longer, and which seem to feature regular posting. A lot of people start groups, which is very easy, and then never do anything else with them.

It's a good idea to get the feel of a group for a day or two before posting, by reading what people are already saying. Think of it as a conversation that you are joining because you just walked into the room. You're bursting with information you want to share, but somebody else is talking, so you are polite and shut up for a moment to let them finish.

However, every online disease discussion group is accustomed to the introductory post that begins: "I don't know where to turn and I hope I've come to the right place ..."

Such cries for help will usually be followed up quickly by support from existing members, who may ask for more information, suggest other more appropriate lists, or offer specific suggestions right off the bat.

Some lists are fully moderated, which means that every post must be approved by somebody in charge before going to the rest of the members. Some lists for medical conditions have affiliated health care professionals available to respond to specific concerns.

Many disease discussion groups are closed, which means that the general public can't see them and you have to be approved by a moderator to join. This is to protect everyone's privacy and sanity. A closed list can prevent the curious, morbid, mean-spirited, or disturbed from showing up and making trouble. These nasty folks are called trolls and you want nothing to do with them or the bridges they live under.

You can get messages from these lists either as they are posted or in daily digest form, wherein all messages throughout the day are sent in a single email. You may also read messages online at the group's homepage, which may include links to other resources. You are not obligated to respond to every email on a list, and if a list isn't working for you, it's easy to unsubscribe.

Many disease websites offer their own online support groups in varying formats. Most will ask for some initial personal information when you join just to verify that you aren't a troll and most have rules of some sorts. Track these leads down as early as you can.

SOCIAL MEDIA

Social media are simple and automatic for younger siblings, and become more problematic as sibling clusters age. In all instances, be very careful not to share *anything* online without your sibling's permission. The Internet is forever. Don't overshare, either. People don't need to know about the results of every lab test.

Facebook is currently the most commonly used social medium for people over fifty. Apart from status updates, you may be able to find special Facebook groups aimed at people confronting the same medical issues you are. Plug your sibling's current medical situation into the Facebook search block where you'd normally put the name of the guy you had a crush on in high school, and you will probably come up with multiple Facebook pages. Some may be local and/or useful.

If you aren't comfortable on social media, learn to be careful about privacy settings so that you don't inadvertently disclose information about your sibling's condition. If you post something on a page with poor privacy settings, others could see the post in their feed and get a lot of details you didn't mean to share outside of what you thought was a limited group. If you have no idea what this means, ask somebody who does know.

PATIENT INFORMATION
DATA-SHARING

One of the most exciting and useful data-sharing groups is not precisely a support group. Patients Like Me (www.patientslikeme.com/) was founded in 2004 by engineers who had just spent five years trying to get information about ALS for a sibling and friend with the disease. They wanted a way to compare medical information and experiences with others in similar situations.

The result is science for, by, and about the masses—a cooperative community where members track their own illnesses, symptoms and treatment regimens and share data with others in similar situations. You can find out what other treatments are currently in use, track personal treatments, and learn about clinical trials that may be exactly what you're looking for. Caregivers are welcome as well.

Patient members may disguise identity to a fair degree and few members have chosen the public option, but the site is based on the notion of sharing, so it has both a privacy policy and an openness policy. They are equally complicated.

Patients Like Me has 200,000 members, so the odds of finding useful information are pretty good.

WHERE DID ALL THOSE BOOKS
COME FROM?

Nobody knows exactly how many different books are loose in the world, but millions of titles are available through Amazon.com, the reigning 500-pound gorilla in the bookselling room. The vast majority of the new books currently available in this Brave New E-Reader World are self-published, which is both a good and a bad thing.

Good in that there is more information available on more topics.

Bad in that these books are often unedited, literally dumped onto the Internet by authors about whom you know nothing beyond what they claim about themselves. Nobody has really vetted most of these books or their authors.

Keep in mind that in the world of contemporary information, the key is Caveat Emptor. *Buyer Beware.*

BUYING BOOKS

If you are in the habit of buying books, you probably have some fairly well-established habits. You may pick them up at the big box store while you're stocking up on gallons of spaghetti sauce and cords of Q-tips. You may snag paperbacks at the drug store or grocery. You may automatically click on your favorite big online bookseller or download books onto your e-reader. You may select something that sounds vaguely familiar at the airport when your flight is delayed due to bad weather in Minneapolis.

You may even go to an actual bookstore.

This is not as easy as it used to be. Independent bookstores are an endangered species, largely driven out of business by high discounts offered through online booksellers, big box outlets, and e-books downloaded directly from the Internet. I personally regard this as a national tragedy, and miss those wonderful places, which featured knowledgeable staff, carefully selected inventory, and occasionally a cat sleeping in a sunny spot in the window.

It is small comfort that the wave of giant bookstores which signaled the demise of so many independent booksellers has now itself imploded. Crown is gone. Borders is out of business. Barnes and Noble is closing stores.

So at a time when there are more book titles available than people living in Denmark or Norway, there are actually fewer places to buy those books. A lot fewer.

There are still a few independent bookstores where you can stand in front of a selection of new titles on the subject which interests you and make a selection after physically examining different choices. These places will happily order anything in print and available through a wholesaler for you, as will the remaining big box bookstores. You can find them at www.indiebound.org.

But nearly all the action today is on the Internet.

SOME BOOKS ARE BETTER THAN OTHER BOOKS

Who can you believe? Who *should* you believe?

Recent books from publishers and/or authors with names that you recognize are generally a safe bet and often are available at the public library. They may be written by medical figures who are familiar from TV news and/or talk shows or by experts with distinguished credentials. Neither is a guarantee, of course, since publishing is both a crapshoot and a part of the free enterprise system. A book may become a bestseller for reasons that defy logic or credibility.

With a major publisher, you know some things for sure: At least one salaried editor at that house read the book, discussed it with the marketing department, thought a particular group of readers would find it interesting enough to purchase, paid the most paltry possible advance to the writer (exception: recently shamed or retired figures from the worlds of entertainment and government) and nursed it through the nine-month gestation period required to produce most hardcover or trade paperback books.

If you're not familiar with the author or title or brand (examples: the Johns Hopkins Hospital series on diseases or the familiar Dummies black-and-yellow covers), you can tell a certain amount by looking more closely at the book itself or at its listing on such major Internet sale sites as Amazon.com.

When was the book published? The publication date is found on the back side of the book's title page at the front of the book and should also appear in any online listing. The more recent the better, particularly for medical information. Instructions on building a wheelchair ramp may not change much over time, but 21st Century medicine moves swiftly. A twenty-year-old disease book might be no more useful than one written during the Middle Ages suggesting leeches or a good bleeding down at the barber shop.

The exception to the age rule is a book first published a while ago and then re-issued subsequently in updated editions. Any book which has gone through several editions will probably be useful, so long as the edition you're using was updated within the past few years.

Are there reviews for the book? Do these come from publications you recognize? A positive review from an industry outlet such as *Publisher's Weekly, Booklist,* or *Library Journal* is a very good sign, as is almost anything from a newspaper or magazine you're familiar with. It is extraordinarily difficult to get any book reviewed by major media today.

If there are reviews from readers, look at them. Do they all say "Best book ever written" or do they appear to be written by real people who actually read the book, addressing their specific concerns?

Advance praise for books, known as blurbs in the publishing world, can be helpful if the praise is specific and comes from people who know something about the subject. If a book about heart disease has blurbs from cardiologists at UCLA and the Mayo Clinic, for example, you're probably on the right track. If the ingénue from your favorite sitcom gushes that it is fabulous, it may only mean that her uncle back home wrote the book.

Many books are only available as e-books, and to read them you'll need to download them onto an electronic device such as a tablet or an e-reader like a Kindle or Nook. You may already have one of these or have access to one. In a pinch, you can download e-books directly to your computer or even a smartphone.

Print publications are usually available both new and used, in a wide range of prices and sizes. Make decisions that are right for you. You are under no obligation to purchase a new copy of a fifteen-pound doorstop that costs eighty-nine bucks and includes a lot of incomprehensible charts, just because it was written by a noted authority.

PROWLING AROUND THE INTERNET

The more specific you make the subject of your search, the more likely you are to find useful information.

Google "breast cancer" and you'll get 237,000,000 hits, which is nearly 237 million more than you have time to check. Google "breast cancer treatment" and you whittle it down to 48 million. Make that "breast cancer lumpectomy" and you're down to 1.32 million. "Tamoxifen after lumpectomy" gets you down to 213,000, and putting quotes around those three words in your search makes it 71,000. Which is still too many.

Don't be afraid to look beyond the top listings in a search, or even the first several pages. I have found some really valuable resources four pages into Google search results. Top listings, particularly for diseases with pricey treatments, are often the result of paid placement and may or may not be obvious ads. Indeed, once you look up a disease on an Internet search engine, your screen will fill with disease-related ads. Often these will be for hospitals or medical groups that would like to be your health care providers. Sometimes they will also be for law firms, if something about an affliction has currently placed it in the litigation arena.

This can, of course, also be a useful way to find local medical specialists, or at least to learn who in your sibling's area believes they are pretty good at treating her disease.

A SECOND WORD OF CAUTION

Not all foundations or disease-related organizations are legitimate. Just because something has a spiffy website doesn't mean it is worth your time or your money.

The Tampa Bay Times compiles an annual list of the fifty worst charities in terms of the amount spent on solicitation and fundraising costs instead of research or education. (www.tampabay.com/americas-worst-charities) Many of these nasty organizations have names which are very similar to legitimate charities that do good works responsibly. Check this list and make sure that you're supporting organizations that spend donations on education, research, and direct aid, instead of paying the guys in the telemarketing boiler room.

YET ANOTHER WORD OF CAUTION

The Internet is constantly changing, rather like the giant blob that rolls down Main Street in a Fifties horror movie, picking up mailboxes and dumping out the occasional small pet as it passes by. People are likely to simply abandon old websites, which will still come up in a search even though they are hopelessly out of date.

The Internet is forever. Right or wrong, current or obsolete.

SERIES BOOKS ON
DISEASES AND CONDITIONS

A number of excellent series of books on diseases and conditions are published by prominent hospitals and medical schools. Some go into greater depth and are far more technical than others, and you may run across some medical school textbooks, which you will probably want to avoid unless you are a doctor yourself.

Libraries often carry some of the more expensive and comprehensive titles, which may turn out to be more information than you need or want anyway. It's up to you to decide just how much you really want to know about Wellington's Wallop.

My favorite series for learning the basics about almost any medical-related topic is the Harvard Medical School Special Health Reports, and sometimes I find that's really all the information I need on a subject (www.health.harvard.edu/special-health-reports). The Health Reports are magazine-type publications that run from 40-50 pages and there are about six dozen of them.

They cover medical problems (Sensitive Gut, Headache, Pain Relief); issues (Change Made Easy, Grief and Loss); mental health and illness; exercise; and pretty much any other health topic from Addiction to Weight Control. Twelve are also available in Spanish. You can download them immediately as PDFs or wait for a copy to be mailed, which is nicer but always seems to take too long.

What I like about them is that they provide solid, basic information in whatever format works best for the topic. Exercises for joint pain are photographed, drugs commonly prescribed for a condition are analyzed and compared in charts, caregiving tips are provided where appropriate. The language is clear and understandable, but technical enough.

OLDER AND OUT-OF-PRINT BOOKS

Older books may have good information as well, and some have become classics. *The 36-Hour Day,* often cited as the quintessential Alzheimer's caregiving book, was first published in 1981 and is currently in its fifth edition.

Many other books may have been traditionally published and then gone out of print, which means that nobody—not you, not your local bookstore, not even the President of the United States—can order new copies from the publisher or from traditional wholesalers any more. Newly-published books go out of print faster and more frequently than most authors are willing to admit, with a shelf life somewhere between milk and yogurt.

The good news for buyers is that you can buy secondhand books easily on the Internet, and the bad news for authors is that at this point all profits go to the person peddling the used volume.

Used books can be ordered several different ways. Great big booksellers such as Amazon or Barnes and Noble also list used books sold by others through their websites. Fewer people are aware of help-the-world bookselling operations like Better World Books or consortiums like my personal favorite, AbeBooks. Links to all—as well as to BooksPrice.com, which compares prices on different sites—are at the end of this chapter.

Better World Books mostly sells library discards, paying a modest amount back to the libraries and donating a portion of their ultimate profits, as well as lots of books, to good causes. Because they carry many library discards (in addition to plenty of civilian stock), you're likely to find fairly recent books on all kinds of diseases, the sort of titles that libraries update and replace frequently.

AbeBooks and other bookselling consortiums serve as a clearing house for thousands of independent booksellers, and make it easy for you to select among them in all sorts of ways. For research, I generally start out with the cheapest and upgrade from there if necessary. I've ordered dozens of books this way and love the simplicity of the system.

AN ECONOMIC SIDE NOTE

If you're going to be ordering books or much of anything online that is sibling-related, you might want to get a separate credit card for those purchases. This makes it easier to keep track should you need the information later, even if you're pretty sure right now that you won't.

I also encourage everybody to have one card that is used only for Internet purchases. That way when your account is hacked—and odds are that it will be—you can have the credit card company issue a new card.

Then you start using that one newly-issued only for online purchases, and so on and so on.

ADDITIONAL INFORMATION

Health Care Systems

Elizabeth Askin & Nathan Moore
The Health Care Handbook: A Clear and Concise Guide to the United States Health Care System
Washington University School of Medicine, 2012

Shannon Brownlee
Overtreated: Why Too Much Medicine is Making Us Sicker and Poorer
Bloomsbury, 2008

Alan Cassels
Seeking Sickness: Medical Screening and the Misguided Hunt for Disease
Greystone, 2012

Rosemary Gibson and Janardan Prasad Singh
The Treatment Trap: How the Overuse of Medical Care is Wrecking Your Health and What You Can Do to Prevent It
Ivan R. Dee, 2011

Lee Gutkind and Pagan Kennedy
An Immense New Power to Heal: The Promise of Personalized Medicine
In Fact Books, 2012

Nancy Snyderman
Medical Myths That Can Kill You: And the 101 Truths that will Save, Extend and Improve Your Life
Three Rivers Press, 2009

H. Gilbert Welch, Lisa M. Schwartz, and Steven Woloshin
Overdiagnosed: Making People Sick in the Pursuit of Health
Beacon Press, 2012

Support Groups

AACR: American Association for Cancer Research (Search for "How to Find a Support Group")
www.aacr.org
866.423.3965

Cancer Support Community (formerly The Wellness Community and Gilda's Club Worldwide)
www.cancersupportcommunity.org
888.793.9355

Facebook
www.facebook.com

Google Groups
www.groups.google.com

MD Junction: People Helping People
www.mdjunction.com/

Mental Health America
www.mentalhealthamerica.net/go/find_support_group

My Cancer Circle: Cancer Support Community for Patients and Caregivers
www.mycancercircle.lotsahelpinghands.com

Patients Like Me: Health Data Sharing
www.patientslikeme.com/

Sharecare (a wide range of diseases, problems, and conditions)
www.dailystrength.org/support-groups

SupportGroups.com
www.supportgroups.com/

Yahoo Groups
www.groups.yahoo.com

Online Sources for New and Second-Hand Books

Independent Booksellers Association – www.indiebound.org
AbeBooks – www.abebooks.com
Amazon.com – www.amazon.com
Barnes and Noble – www.bn.com
Better World Books – www.betterworldbooks.com
Bookfinder.com –www.bookfinder.com
BooksPrice.com – www.booksprice.com (compares prices on different websites)

TEN THINGS NOT TO DO

In the course of any sibling relationship there are times when what you don't do is even more important than what you do. This dates back to when you knew better than to give your toddler brother a Milk-Bone for a snack, or to tell your older sister that her prom dress made her look like a frilly lampshade at Kitsch-o-Rama.

We're all older now, and possibly a bit wiser. Your family is dealing with a situation that everybody hoped would never occur—if they thought of the possibility at all. It's rough. But as you attempt to move forward, let me remind you of a few things that aren't likely to help and could make matters a good deal worse.

1. Don't be judgmental.

It's entirely possible that you always knew better, but this isn't the time to make a big deal out of it.

Maybe your sister was a smoker, or overweight. Maybe she didn't exercise enough or exercised too much. She may have delayed getting medical help while ignoring symptoms and hoping they would go away. She might have been a little casual about following doctors' orders. She may have been blowing a 1.3 when she smashed into a tree.

It isn't necessary to call attention to something that everybody realizes. This is also the wrong moment to impose your own values or try to correct anybody's perceptions about much of anything. A major health crisis requires everybody in the boat to be rowing in the same direction.

This is most particularly not the time to say, "I told you so," even if you have to bite your tongue bloody not to.

What's done is done. *I told you so* was infuriating when you were a child and it's no more palatable now. Somebody whose illness can be attributed to personal weakness or failure almost invariably knows that at some level.

You can't retroactively hold your sibling to your own standards.

This is particularly important if you're somebody who schedules quarterly dental checkups and annual mammograms, squeezes full dollar out of the gym membership and is about to take on a triathlon. You are undoubtedly proud of all this, as you should be. But your siblings may privately find these virtues a colossal pain. They may, indeed, also resent the cloud of moral superiority that those virtues sometimes travel in.

Folks get behind on self-care and preventive health measures, for whatever reasons: fear, money, indifference, or maybe even Iatrophobia, fear of doctors. If your sister is now facing serious consequences from that "forgetfulness," she is well aware of what she should have done differently. Your pointing out the obvious isn't going to help anything.

Particularly if you've always been considered the judgmental one.

2. Don't take over.

Your instinct may be to do this. The very fact that you're involved at all suggests you may have a tendency in this direction.

Resist it.

Take your cues from your sick sibling, at least initially. Is help wanted? Expected? Who initiated your insertion into this health care situation?

If you answered a cry for help—whether from your sibling, your sibling's spouse, or children of any age—that's different. If your sibling is incapacitated, there may be decisions to make or alternatives to consider, and some of these may need to happen pretty quickly.

If you've always been the bossy older sibling it can be very easy to slip into the take-charge mode, but doing so may actually prove counterproductive. Look for areas on which all parties agree and move forward as cautiously as possible from that shared ground.

But also be warned: It's a lot easier to assume

responsibility for something than it is to later relinquish that responsibility, even if everybody is currently making at least an effort to get along and work together.

Don't agree to do something or take charge of something if you aren't comfortable assuming that the responsibility will last for six months or longer.

3. Don't make decisions without sufficient input.

Whose input? Ah, that's the big question, and very case-specific.

If your sister is in a coma or the ICU, it isn't reasonable to expect input from the patient, at least not right away. If she has signed Advance Directives, her wishes have precedence over your own. But if her intentions are *not* spelled out legally, things can get complicated.

If it's early on and decisions don't need to be made immediately, don't make them.

If there *are* issues that must be handled or settled quickly, proceed with caution. These are decisions of the who's-covering-the-light-bill or should-we-consider-hospice sort, not who's going out for sandwiches. You'll be surprised how many things can be put off in the middle of a health emergency, and how generally understanding people can be.

The reality is that this needs to be a team effort, assuming that you've been able to cobble together something resembling a team.

Try not to venture out on shaky health-decision limbs without additional family input, the better to build consensus. If you proceed this way, you're also less likely to have some irritated family member saw off the whole damn branch.

In the face of hotly contested and very important decisions, bring in the outside forces you believe your sister would want involved. This may be her minister, a hospital chaplain, her financial adviser, her lifelong best friend, her business partner, or the neighbor with whom she's had coffee every morning for thirty years.

Listen to these people. They probably know your sister

in ways you never thought of, and possibly a lot better than you know her. But do make it clear that you're the one with decision-making responsibility, and that you're soliciting input, not asking for instruction.

Perhaps her circle is lacking in those types of friends and colleagues, and decision-making seems to keep falling onto you no matter how much you might want to deflect it. In that case, try to decide things the way you think that she would decide them, and be honest about it.

To do this in a logical and reasoned fashion, consult your *own* circle of trusted friends and advisors. These people know how *you* think, what you're reading into the situation, and how best to help you make difficult decisions.

4. Don't get into a pissing match that isn't necessary.

With anybody.

In the early stages of a serious illness, when folks are all riled up about the shock and confusion and horror of the whole situation, it's easy to back yourself into a corner over something that is really pretty inconsequential. Bad idea.

Try to get along as best you can with everybody. And if "everybody" happens to include hospital personnel, it's worth going to extra trouble to be nice to the men and women who are directly involved with the care of your brother.

You can't be there around the clock, but the relationship you establish with caregivers will be.

5. Don't let the past get in the way of the present.

Whatever slights, differences, arguments, or world-class fights you and your siblings may have left floating in the family biosphere, now is the time to let them go and concentrate on what you are all hoping to accomplish for your ailing sibling. If this requires a sit-down, then arrange a meeting for the parties involved. If something truly awful once happened and it is not in the "forgivable" category, either figure out a way to set it aside, or excuse whoever was involved from current participation.

The present will be difficult enough without letting yourselves be eaten alive by your past.

6. Don't foist your religious beliefs on people who don't already agree with you.

To every thing there is a season, and the season to proselytize is not when you're dealing with a medical crisis.

Your beliefs are your own, and your siblings may believe things that are altogether different. Your family may, indeed, represent a veritable smorgasbord of spiritual beliefs. Now is not the time to point out the error of your siblings' ways, to bring in unwelcome clergy, or to make a giant fuss about anything that isn't directly related to life-or-death issues.

If that feels too hard to handle, pray on it.

7. Don't force new technology on somebody who doesn't want it.

If your ailing brother is a computer luddite with advanced disinterest in all things electronic, this isn't the time to show him the error of his ways. Maybe later, when he feels better.

This is also true of those in the circle you may be building to share caregiving and other responsibilities. If you are the only one who knows the difference between a URL and the Early Warning System, it won't help anything if you devise a really clever online caregiving schedule.

By all means use your own expertise in any way that will be helpful, including research, but tailor other assignments and digital expectations to your audience.

8. Don't try to be Superman or Wonder Woman.

You can't do everything. It's just that simple.

So don't try.

If you make yourself sick, you're not helping anybody and you may be setting matters back. Pace yourself. Stop and take deep breaths. Go for a walk around the block. Drink a glass of orange juice when you get back.

When you're in a particularly challenging situation of any sort, it can seem overwhelming. So concentrate on dealing with its more manageable aspects, one little piece at a time.

9. Don't try to solve the unsolvable.

Sometimes problems can't be solved. Sometimes they can barely be addressed.

If you find yourself in a situation where even the most solid ground is a quagmire, you are not obligated to get yourself in neck deep before conceding defeat.

However, sometimes problems which appear insurmountable will morph into something altogether different if you ignore them a little while. They may even just go away. In a fast-breaking medical situation, there's actually little advantage in trying to stay very far ahead of the curve, because you really don't know which way it's going to break, or when.

Still, even though you usually don't know the dimensions of the SibCare box when you first discover you're in it, it helps to try to think outside that box.

Inspiration may strike when you least expect it.

10. Don't second-guess yourself.

Ever.

SECTION THREE:

PAPERWORK

THE PAPERWORK MORASS:
Personal, Medical, Financial

Almost everybody dislikes paperwork. For many folks it is a visceral hatred that's one part childhood homework memories, one part monthly bill-paying, and one huge part whatever-is-required-in-the-way-of-paperwork-on-the-job.

In a SibCare situation, you'll be dealing with different kinds of paperwork. Current incoming is whatever the mail brings from this day forward, along with medical paperwork generated during doctor and treatment visits. Past incoming and outgoing may need to be organized and dealt with, especially if there are unpaid bills or if there's confusion about medical matters. And finally, there are documents that haven't been created yet but need to be. Many of these will be covered in the next chapter on "Legal Paperwork."

It's easy to put off a lot of what we'll discuss here, unless you have a major ongoing medical or financial emergency. This is not smart. If you don't have the appropriate paperwork in place, you can find yourself in a world of trouble when your family turns an unforeseen medical corner.

Plunging into the paperwork morass, you may feel a bit like those brave souls who take a New Year's Day swim with the Polar Bear Club. It's cold out there, and scary. Also, plowing through, digging out, organizing, creating, and otherwise beating paperwork into submission is generally a pretty lonely and solitary venture.

If it promises to be a huge task, try to find somebody you trust who can work with you. This may feel like an invasion of privacy, but the reality is that severe illness obliterates all kinds of privacy, and matters will only get worse if you don't find a way to get on top of them. Be sure that your assistant understands confidentiality, of course.

If the mere thought of all this sends you into a frenzy, a good place to start is with the website Get Your Shit Together (GYST). Don't be put off by the less-than-felicitous name. This site is a mission of mercy, created by a woman who was not yet forty when her husband was killed in an accident. To help others avoid the frustration and anxiety she experienced trying to figure out things she never dreamed she'd need to know, she created GYST. We are all the richer for her generosity.

GYST has templates for many of the paperwork projects you'll need to confront and control, and all are downloadable for free. The legal documents tend to be based on Washington state, however, which is only a good idea if you live in Washington state. Every state has its own specific (and occasionally arcane) legal requirements, which will also be discussed in "Legal Paperwork."

This may already feel a bit overwhelming, but just about anyone can benefit from downloading the GYST Details template to get started. You can also sign up to receive gentle quarterly reminders to GYST. These are particularly useful if you are not dealing with an emergency, or if you have your sibling's affairs in order but you need to do the same thing for yourself. www.getyourshittogether.org/

IF PAPERWORK IS IN DISARRAY

Okay, *disarray* is a euphemism.

I'm not talking about a single envelope slightly misaligned on an otherwise immaculate home desk. I'm talking about the kind of situation where random piles of paper are toppling over while other piles have been crammed into drawers and boxes. Where you don't have a clue how to identify and locate what you need, or pay what needs to be paid, or determine what has been happening and why.

First and foremost, don't panic.

When I went to help my brother after his first stroke, he'd been in the hospital and rehab for three weeks. Before that, he had labored valiantly to deal with escalating financial problems. One table was set up with a calculator and IRS materials and tax records. Another had neatly piled medical bills and Explanations of Benefits. And the dining table and chairs were overflowing with recently-arrived envelopes covered with red ink and dire warnings.

In this case, where to start was easy. I got the phone turned on again. I also decided not to even listen to the three dozen messages on the answering machine because I didn't have the time or stomach for them. Turned out they were all from bill collectors anyway. *Quelle surprise.*

If somebody has been building up to a major medical problem, everyday affairs sometimes don't get handled in a timely manner. For others, of course, this also happens in perfect health. You know who you are.

If you are thrust into a situation where you need to deal with a paperwork jungle, take a deep breath and treat it as an archeological dig. **Don't throw anything away until you are certain you don't need it.**

Last week's grocery flyer can go, but anything that says URGENT or SECOND NOTICE or IMMEDIATE ACTION NEEDED should have top priority. Hang on to anything you aren't sure of. This is the stage when you can easily toss something that will be crucial later, though once you are aware of the existence of a report or bill or whatever, you can generally get a new copy.

The most current and pressing matters are likely to be near the top. This includes current and past due utility bills, credit card statements, mortgage and rent payments, medical co-pays, insurance premiums, and so on.

Begin with a basic triage and separate things into broad general categories. It can help to get some small and medium-sized clear plastic bins for this sorting. Useful categories to start with are Household Bills, Credit Cards, Medical, Receipts,

Personal. As others become obvious, start new bins. Fold a piece of paper in half and write each category name on it in marker, then drape the ID over the side of the bin so it's easy to read. You may think you'll remember what's what, but it's always easier with labels. Always.

If it turns out that there is a lot more of one thing than you expected (ideally uncashed checks rather than unpaid bills), move it into a bigger bin and switch the ID paper to that container. When you have everything (or at least everything that seems current) divided into categories, you can then slide each folded ID paper into the side of the box, print side out, and put its lid on. Then you can easily identify the contents without having to open the box. This process of closing up the box is psychologically useful if you are dealing with a lot of different problems at once.

Even as you work to bring past paper into order, make sure you have identified one place where new paper goes as it comes in. Always. Immediately. No exceptions. This can be as simple as a basket by the front door.

If you are being hounded by bill collectors, put them all off at first by announcing that your sibling is very ill, with elaboration as you see fit (in ICU, had a stroke, undergoing chemotherapy, whatever fits). We'll talk more about bill collectors later.

CREATING A PERSONAL DOSSIER

As soon as possible, you should begin creating a Personal Dossier of information for and about your sibling.

This information doesn't need to be widely distributed, nor should it be, but it must be complete, current, and available in one place for those who need it. Start with the patient's name, address, phone, email, date of birth, and Social Security number. Make photocopies of Social Security, insurance, and Medicare/Medicaid cards, along with copies of passport, driver's license and/or state ID card. Include organ donor information if relevant. Put all this in a file folder or expandable file.

If your sibling doesn't have a state-issued ID of some sort, make every effort to get one as soon as possible. This is usually handled through the state Department of Motor Vehicles.

Any time that you add something to the Dossier, include the appropriate phone numbers, websites, and login information (generally user names and passwords, sometimes with security questions about first pets, etc.) for any associated websites. This may include insurance, Medicare or Medicaid, doctor's offices, mail order pharmacies, etc. Don't worry if this gets messy, or if you are simply slipping pieces of paper into the file. The important part is that you are gathering it in one place.

You should also include military records; marriage and divorce records with dates; residency, citizenship and naturalization papers if applicable; and copies of legal documents that deal with specific situations. When you generate more legal documents, add them to the file.

As you gather information, think in terms of what you'll need to know to access something related to it. Write down names, addresses, email addresses and phone numbers, and include any numbers associated with the account or organization or whatever.

Of course you'll be gathering information about relevant health insurance, but don't forget other types of insurance people carry: automobile, homeowner's or renter's, excess, life, disability, long-term care. Get names, addresses, and numbers for all of these, and if you are involved in bill paying, figure out what the payment cycle is.

If you have time to type this all up neatly and print extra copies, all the better.

When working on the Dossier, remember that you are much better off having too much information than being one crucial item short somewhere down the line.

MEDICATION LIST

This gets included in the Personal Dossier, but it will also be used elsewhere.

The patient's name, address, and phone number go at the top of the sheet. If there are drug allergies, note them clearly. Then list exactly what your sibling takes, with dosages and times. Include any and all vitamins, supplements, herbs, and/or miracle cures that may be on the current menu. Make a note of the pharmacies that are normally used, both local and mail-order, with phone numbers and websites. If medications are ordered from out of the country, make sure that the mechanism for that is also clear.

At the bottom of the sheet list the primary care physician's name and number, along with contact info for any other specialists currently in play (oncologist, radiologist, orthopedist, surgeon, etc.). Finish it off with contact information for you and any other relatives or caregivers who should be notified in case of emergency.

Make plenty of copies of this and see that they are readily available: taped inside the medicine cabinet or on the bathroom mirror, on the refrigerator (particularly useful if paramedics arrive and need information in a hurry), in your sibling's purse or wallet, and in *your* purse or wallet.

Take a copy along to every medical visit, particularly if you are dealing with multiple health care providers. When one doctor prescribes something, the others need to know about it. That helps avoid prescribing things that may cancel out each other's beneficial effects or, even worse, trigger a negative reaction.

MEDICAL HISTORY

This doesn't need to include every hangnail since puberty, but it should list any surgical procedures, major illnesses, hospitalizations, specialized treatments such as radiation and chemotherapy—and the various diagnoses associated with these.

If there has been a misdiagnosis along the way (perhaps with some ineffective treatment attached) note that as well. Dates aren't critical so long as they are reasonably close. It doesn't matter whether your sister was 32 or 34 when she had gall bladder surgery, but it is more important to list that operation than the precise date she broke her toe.

If your sibling can work with you to put this together, all the better. If the cooperation level is not what it might be, do as much as possible on your own and then ask for help on things you're not sure of.

If your sibling isn't able to help at all, do the best you can with available records and memories. By the time my brother needed assistance from his sisters, his cumulative brain damage allowed no clear concept of dates and specific incidents beyond his original treatment fourteen years earlier.

He did, however, have a ton of files devoted to those fourteen years. I hauled home a suitcase full of paper and created a detailed history from it. That history was more complex than anybody needed, actually, and for all I know it missed some stuff altogether. But it gave us all something to work from.

It was also particularly useful when he'd start over with a new set of doctors in a new location, which happened four times in as many years.

MEDICAL NOTEBOOK

Use the medications list and history to start a medical notebook. Numerous medical organizing notebooks are available commercially, but you can also simply set up your own, just like the notebooks you carried in grade school.

Your tabs will say Medications and Lab Reports instead of Math and Reading, but it's the same principle. Include some dividers with pockets so you can stash lab reports or prescriptions, and if the notebook really starts to grow, invest in a three-hole punch to keep it current and easy to access.

Modify this notebook to meet your specific needs. If there are certain things you are closely monitoring (blood pressure, weight, heart rate, levels of whatever), set up a special section for that information, with whatever charts you may need to fill in.

A medical notebook can also be easily expanded to include caregiver notes and scheduling information if multiple family members are involved or professional caregivers have been hired.

MASTER CALENDAR

You can make this fancy, but you don't need to. Set up at least one place where all appointments and scheduled events will be automatically listed. It can be the kitchen calendar, a day planner, an electronic device synched to other electronic devices, or some combination of these. Just be sure that everybody knows about it and that every upcoming appointment and event gets recorded immediately.

SHARING INFORMATION

If the people on your sibling's care team are computer savvy, the easiest way to track, update, and share all this information may be through an app or website such as Dropbox, Evernote, or a similar cloud-based service.

If you are dealing with a lower level of digital sophistication, telephone or email will also work fine. Just keep in mind that if everybody but one or two luddites is participating in a more advanced system, somebody needs to *always* update them using more traditional methods.

PASSWORDS

Almost everything is password-protected these days.

Make a list of all the passwords that your sibling uses for anything, and keep adding to it as you think of additional items. Some things are obvious: home computer, laptop or tablet, cell phone, email accounts. If he does any social networking, you'll need passwords to access those sites. Online shoppers may have dozens of accounts with different login information, and often that information exists only in their heads.

Savvy techno-people are always warning us to have a different password for every account and to change them regularly to something that looks like **du&3E9*!5qLP**. This is not the place for lectures on digital security, but if you discover that your brother has been using **PASSWORD** or **12345678** for everything, this would probably be a good time to change these to something at least slightly more secure.

Your sibling may not want to share these passwords which are, after all, intended to preserve personal privacy. Be gentle but firm about this. You aren't intending to hijack your sister's Victoria's Secret account, after all, or order up a party and some porn on your brother's MasterCard.

It may help if you point out that this synchronized info will be available for your sibling's own use when recovery is complete and everything is back to normal again.

CONTACTS

Through the course of your sibling's illness, you may find yourself interacting with a lot of different people, none of whom you knew before.

Collect business cards from everybody and keep them in a central location. The easiest way is to put them all in a small, conveniently-located box or basket. Or take two of each and tape the second set to pages in the Medical Notebook. If you have an electronic system for entering contacts, do so. You may not need these folks often (or ever), but it's nice to be able to put your hands on their info when you do.

Make sure that all current health care provider names and numbers are also stored in your phone and your sibling's.

THE FINANCIAL DOSSIER

Your sister may be handling all her financial matters

very capably on her own right now, but at some point in the future that could change. To be prepared, you'll also need to create a Financial Dossier. This should be separate from the personal one.

Set up an easily-accessed file or notebook that includes *all* banking information: accounts, locations, log-in information, PINs. If you are going to be involved in bill-paying or financial management, you need to be a signatory on those accounts, and should also have a Durable Power of Attorney to facilitate using them. This is explained in the chapter called "Legal Paperwork."

Figure out and record all sources of income and when that income arrives. You may need to dig around a bit for this, and it may turn out that your sibling is entitled to something not yet being received—a work pension, for instance, or Social Security.

Credit card information should all be included, including oddball cards that are rarely used. The easiest way to do this is to empty a wallet and photocopy everything on both sides. If credit card accounts are handled online, make sure that all website and login information is current, written down, and accessible.

Many people have some of their bill payments or debt service on auto-payments. They may also be receiving paperless bills. The more you can learn about current financial routines and practices, the less likely you are to have unpleasant surprises. This is true whether or not you are going to be involved in day-to-day financial matters.

Auto-debits can be tricky, particularly if they were set up a long time ago. They are also hard to stop and may require research to even determine what they are.

A friend spent a ridiculous amount of time tracking down six seemingly-simple payments that her father had set up decades earlier for monthly auto-debit from a checking account. All were for some form of life insurance, but by the time she needed the information, several issuing companies no longer existed, having been swallowed by other corporations multiple times. And so on. I'm actually not sure if she ever found them all.

SAFE DEPOSIT BOXES

Safe deposit boxes can be a real pain. If your sibling has one, find out what's kept in it and why. This is *not* the place to keep paperwork that needs to be quickly accessed, such as a will or burial instructions. You most definitely do not want Advance Directives in here because if you need them in a hurry, you'll be totally out of luck.

People often get a safe deposit box for a particular reason and hold on to it long after that reason passes. Then the key gets misplaced, and when somebody tries to gain access later, there are all kinds of legal hassles and maybe also a hefty charge to drill the lock, only to find that the box is empty or contains old Valentines.

Shortly before my brother went to live with his stepdaughter, I discovered an annual auto-debit on his checking account for a safe deposit box I didn't know about. I was 1,800 miles away at the time, but I'd collected dozens of miscellaneous keys on a previous visit and placed them all in a single kitchen drawer. My resourceful niece dumped those keys into a bag, then took the bag and my brother to the bank branch where (we hoped) the box was located. Bank officials were able to identify the key and they opened and cleared out the box, which held nothing essential.

If you can possibly clear up safe deposit box issues now, for heaven's sake do it.

PROPERTY

Property includes real estate, of course—home, vacation home, rental properties, and the one-tenth share of a plot in the middle of nowhere where a group of friends have agreed to meet when the world is coming to an end.

It also includes automobiles, RVs, boats, snowmobiles, ATVs, motorcycles and most large items with wheels. It may include jewelry or valuable collections, artwork, antiques, and items that have greater sentimental value than financial.

Collect the relevant information for any and all of these to include in the Financial Dossier: insurance, registration, maintenance records (and location thereof), and contact information for whoever services or cares for any of these. If there are valuable items that might be overlooked, such as a diamond bracelet tossed in with a lot of costume jewelry, find out where to look for them.

If you know of a particular item of financial or family value and you don't see it anywhere, ask. This is particularly important if you know that your sibling has a tendency to hide things for safekeeping. All too often, folks squirrel things away and then either forget where they hid them or become incapacitated before they can pass on the information. Getting as much info as possible now may help you avoid having to frantically search for something later, hoping and praying it hasn't accidentally been donated to Goodwill.

INVESTMENTS

Compile information for the Financial Dossier on savings accounts; credit unions; stocks, bonds, and other investments; 401(k) and IRA accounts; and any other way that your sibling may have tucked things away for the future. This includes fruit jars buried in the backyard.

Be sure to get sufficient contact information for any individual brokers or bankers who may handle investment matters, and once again list as much basic information as you can find: names and addresses, account numbers, passwords.

BILL PAYING

If you need to get involved in paying your sibling's bills, either temporarily or on a more permanent basis, step back first to assess the overall situation.

Are things in order and up to date? If so, move to the head of the line. All you really need to do here is continue things as they've been handled, or modify them slightly to make matters more convenient for you.

If you're looking at a more complex situation—or one that is a nightmare of past due notices, canceled accounts, and threatening notices—your learning curve is likely to be a lot steeper, and will probably need to start with a Durable Power of Attorney authorizing you to handle financial matters.

Once you've gathered bills that are due or overdue, separate them into categories: household, credit cards, taxes, insurance, medical, other. Do the same thing with sources of income or liquid assets such as savings accounts. You're hoping for sufficient income or resources to cover what is owed on a regular basis, with enough left over for the occasional hot fudge sundae.

What's the monthly nut? How much does it take to keep a roof over your brother's head and the heat and lights on? What other expenses come up quarterly, or semi-annually, or annually? Insurance and property taxes are easy to forget when you're trying to figure out what they call the gas company in his town.

If money is tight and/or income insufficient to meet expenses, look for obvious expenses that can be cut back or eliminated, such as the newspaper nobody's reading or the cable TV package with 1,457 channels. Look for recurring nonessential expenses and let them go. You may need to pay an early cancellation fee, but usually it's worth it.

This may not be as easy as it sounds. After I got my brother's land line turned back on (he had no mobile phone) I took a look at what he was being charged for. There were blocking charges he no longer needed, and a monthly fee for call waiting. A bit of digging revealed that he had been making less than a dozen calls a month and was getting incoming calls only from bill collectors. I decided they could bloody well call back if they got a busy signal, and tried to change his service.

Unsuccessfully.

Because I wasn't already on the account and he was too incapacitated at the moment to authorize me verbally, I got nowhere. I should note here that nobody at AT&T had given a fig who I might be when I gave my own credit card number to turn the service back on only days earlier. But I had bigger fish to fry just then anyway, and let it go. When he was later living on his own again, I encouraged him to call and make the changes, but he had major memory problems, was always put on hold or confronted with a daunting telephone menu, and quickly gave up when he remembered to even try.

If a nonessential service has already been cut off, figure out how much is owed, make a note of it, and then move that bill to the Later pile.

Medical bills can accumulate quickly, particularly if insurance is inadequate or nonexistent. Here you'll want to figure which medical caregivers are involved in current care; they should at least be paid something, as a gesture of good faith. Move any previous care providers who aren't being currently used to the Later pile, though you should be prepared to move them back to Active status if the situation changes.

Credit card bills can expand with frightening speed, and additional charges begin to accumulate like flies on a manure pile. If a monthly minimum payment isn't made, a late charge occurs. At the same time, interest charges are added monthly, including on those late fees, and interest is likely to move to a higher rate while this goes on. This all relates to the Terms and Conditions flyers that are printed in flyspeck and tucked into the bill, filled with language written by attorneys and then translated a few times by Babelfish before coming back to English.

But wait! We're not done. Credit card companies have other tricks. One of my brother's credit card companies lowered his credit limit for nonpayment while all the other charges were piling on, then added additional fees when his balance surpassed that limit.

PUT OUT THE LITTLE FIRES

When you have a lot of creditors clamoring for their pound of flesh, it's hard to know where to start. Sure, you want to keep the heat and lights on, but who comes next?

One trick I learned early was to try to deal with the smaller bills first. I couldn't do that on a regular basis because it took quite a while to get various disability payments into play, but any time a cash infusion appeared, I would pay off a handful of the smaller bills and move them into the Paid file. This provided a huge and unanticipated psychological boost, if for no other reason than that those people were no longer bombarding me with nasty mail.

DEALING WITH CREDITORS

If there are a lot of past due bills, expect to hear from bill collectors, and don't anticipate a lot of sympathy from them. Don't expect them to know that your sister is sick or anything except that there is a bill for a certain amount. For one thing, each time somebody calls from a creditor company or service, it's usually the first time that person has seen the file. So you will need to tell your tale of woe over and over again, no matter how frequently you are talking to Big Unfeeling Corporation representatives.

If anything, this gets worse when a bill is sent to a collection agency, which will be paid a percentage of whatever they can recover from a creditor in arrears.

If you have read this far and are still tearing out your hair, get hold of one or more of the references on credit problems listed at the end of the chapter, many published by the exceptionally trustworthy Nolo Press. I could have saved myself a world of anxiety—and a lot of time—if I'd known to do that. www.nolo.com

The National Foundation for Credit Counseling (NFCC) can direct you to a local credit counselor who will work with you for little or nothing to determine just what kind of situation your sibling is in. In some cases, they may be able to help you work out a Debt Management Plan (DMP) through the local credit counseling agency. Monthly payments to the agency are apportioned to creditors, over a period of 36-60 months.

Initial contact with the NFCC is only by phone, at

800-682-9832. Additional information is available at the website. www.nfcc.org

The Patient Advocate Foundation can provide assistance with medical debt issues, especially if they are related to underinsurance or lack of insurance. www.patientadvocate.org

THE IRS

One very specific type of debt is past due income taxes, and this is a place where it is wise to get professional assistance. If your sibling already has a problematic relationship with the Internal Revenue Service, you'll be well served to get a tax professional involved.

You can't ignore the IRS, tempting though that may be, and bankruptcy won't necessarily discharge an income tax obligation. It is possible to deal directly with them, but I employed an Enrolled Agent, somebody who had retired into private practice after 25 years as an IRS agent.

She was able to determine what my brother actually owed and was obligated to pay and which returns should be amended because he had made errors or omissions that favored the government. She understood deadlines and statutes of limitations, where each form or piece of paper should be sent, and what could and couldn't be done. Eventually she worked out a payment plan that allowed him to retire the debt honorably over time, without paying one penny more than he owed.

You do not necessarily need a CPA for this, though if you already have a good working relationship with your own tax professional, that may be the easiest way to handle matters. You may be able to get by just fine with an Enrolled Agent, and you can find one at the National Association of Enrolled Agents. www.naea.org. Just don't expect to take a banker's box full of papers into a storefront office in March and have a seasonal tax preparer fix things up.

LET'S MAKE A DEAL

If you are trying to retire a specific, non-recurring debt, you may be able to work out an arrangement with the creditor. They might be willing to accept a smaller amount if you can pay it all at once so that everybody can be done with it. Or they might be willing to set up a payment plan for the full or a reduced amount over a prolonged period of time.

If you manage to do this before a debt is turned over to collection, all the better. A collection agency will charge the creditor for squeezing money out of you, but most creditors prefer to get the money directly rather than to share it.

This is a particularly useful technique for dealing with small businesses or medical offices that are overwhelmed by the paperwork involved in collections. It's always worth a try, and even if it doesn't work out, you have demonstrated your desire to deal with this financial obligation in good faith.

CONSUMER RIGHTS

It may not seem like it when you're fielding dunning calls from people who show no apparent interest in your sibling's health or well-being, but the consumer does have quite a few rights. If finances are a mess, learn these rights.

The Fair Debt Collection Practices Act sets out very clear limitations on acceptable behavior by creditors: who can call, when and where, what can be said and what can't be said. Various methods of threatening are specifically addressed and forbidden. If you find yourself in this situation, the FDCPA is your new BFF. Learn the terms and legal limitations that it covers and pay attention to what creditors do and don't say. If they step over the line, nail them.

www.consumer.ftc.gov/articles/0149-debt-collection

BANKRUPTCY

If things are truly a mess, it may be necessary to file for bankruptcy.

This is not a decision that can be made until you've gone through all the assets and liabilities, but if you are trying to make things balance and it looks hopeless, keep it in the back of your mind.

If you believe that it isn't going to be possible to fix your sibling's finances, avoid the kind of bill consolidation services that advertise on late night TV. Talk to a bankruptcy attorney instead. Visit a couple if it makes you feel better, and find somebody you are comfortable with. As a general rule, an initial consultation is free.

When this appeared to be my brother's only option, I met with an attorney who gave me a detailed packet of paperwork to be completed before anything could be done. Oddly, the simple fact of addressing that paperwork gave me more confidence that we could somehow make matters work.

And we did. Eventually it was possible to pay off everybody he owed.

ONLINE BILL PAYING

The easiest way to manage bill payment for somebody else is to have the bills directed to you at your own snail mail or email address and to pay them online from a checking account on which you are a signatory. Changing a billing address is relatively easy and can usually be done online, whether you are using an account for a creditor that your sibling has already set up or creating a new one.

If you are paying bills online for somebody else, you should have a Durable Power of Attorney. And if this makes your sibling uneasy, point out that it can be rescinded anytime. You might also mention that when you personally step back out of the picture later, everything will be set up and humming, just waiting for him to take charge.

I hadn't used online bill payment before it was suggested by an officer at my brother's bank when we had my Durable Power of Attorney signed and notarized. I was initially wary, but quickly discovered I liked the system so much that I also set up my personal bills to be paid online. This can be done on a company-by-company basis, or through the bank's own bill paying service. I use a combination of the two.

You may need to pay bills a couple of times a month if the due dates don't all come together neatly. In some cases, you can change due dates for regular monthly bills, or payment schedules for stuff that's only due a few times a year. Something paid monthly may be easier to keep track of than a quarterly auto insurance payment or an annual homeowner's insurance bill. If money is not an immediate problem, however, you may want to pay these less often, but in full.

ADDITIONAL INFORMATION

Credit Repair Kit
Nolo Press
www.nolo.com/products/credit-repair-kit-pr114.html

Get Your Shit Together
www.getyourshittogether.org

National Association of Enrolled Agents
www.naea.org
855.880.NAEA (6232)

National Foundation for Credit Counseling (NFCC)
www.nfcc.org/index.cfm
800.682.9832

Patient Advocate Foundation
www.patientadvocate.org
800.532.5274

Pension Rights Center
www.pensionrights.org/
888.420.6550

• • • • •

Ken Clark
The Complete Idiot's Guide to Getting Out of Debt
ALPHA, 2009

Melanie Cullen and Shae Irving
Get it Together: Organize Your Records So Your Family Won't Have To, 5th Edition
Nolo, 2012

Stephen Elias
The New Bankruptcy: Will it Work for You?, 4th Edition
Nolo, 2011

Brandi Funk
Cut Your Health Care Costs Now!
CreateSpace, 2010

Bethany K. Laurence and Stephen Elias
Bankruptcy for Small Business Owners: How to File for Chapter 7, 17th Edition
Nolo, 2011

Kathleen Michon and Stephen Elias
Chapter 13 Bankruptcy: Keep Your Property and Repay Debts Over Time, 11th Edition
Nolo, 2012

Margaret Reiter and Robin Leonard
Solve Your Money Troubles: Debt, Credit & Bankruptcy: 13th Edition
Nolo, 2011

Margaret Reiter and Robin Leonard
Credit Repair, 10th Edition
Nolo, 2011

Albin Renauer, Robin Leonard, and Stephen Elias
How to File for Chapter 7 Bankruptcy, 17th Edition, Nolo, 2011

LEGAL PAPERWORK

In a serious medical situation, it is impossible to avoid legal paperwork. Everywhere a patient turns there are releases to be signed and authorizations to be updated—and that's just the day-to-day stuff.

For the longer term, there are several other very important legal documents that every adult should have. Yes, every single one, including you, your children, and your friends.

These documents are confusing to almost everyone, and this chapter will try to de-mystify this legal paperwork and clarify why it's important. That way you can help your sibling be properly papered for whatever may be coming.

Different levels of legal paperwork serve different needs at different times. The more of them that you can get into place early on, the easier things will be for you later.

It may actually help to have a blizzard of paperwork to sign and file all at once, particularly if you are working with a sibling who is less than fully cooperative. Then you can make light of how you're handling everything at one time even though it won't be necessary for decades.

It may also help get your sib's cooperation if you and other family members are completing the same paperwork at the same time. Nobody *wants* to think they'll need this stuff, but when you need it, you really need it. This will create a twofer: setting a good example while covering your own tail.

In a perfect world, your sister will have already met with a certified estate planning attorney and will have drawn up paperwork to cover every possible situation. The attorney will have originals and copies will be available for whoever needs to use them whenever.

Alas, this is rarely a perfect world.

DO YOU NEED A LAWYER?

The answer to this will depend on who you ask.

Those in the legal profession will say that yes, of course, you absolutely do. However, there are plenty of very good resources available to the lay person and you may find that these will meet your needs quite well enough.

If money is not a significant issue, you may choose the comfort of working one-on-one with an attorney, somebody whose job and training it is to prepare estate planning materials.

This is not the time to use your neighbor's kid who just got out of law school or your friend's cousin who practices criminal law. You want somebody who works in the estate planning field, or who at least comes highly recommended by somebody for whom similar paperwork has already been prepared. The attorney should be licensed in the state where your sibling lives, because everything related to this type of legal paperwork is state-specific.

When I first became involved in my brother's care, I was traveling 1800 miles with almost no clue what I was getting into. But I did know that his legal paperwork was woefully out of date and that there was a good chance that he had once completed it with his now ex-wife as beneficiary. Just because he didn't have that paperwork accessible didn't mean that it wasn't going to show up later. I was able to use that threat to leverage him into some movement.

Which makes this an excellent time to point out that you can use worst case scenario threats to get your sibling to cooperate in the paperwork venture if necessary. Threaten, cajole, or plead. Cry if necessary. Just get it done.

For my brother, I was able to handle all the requisite legal paperwork using inexpensive *Quicken WillMaker* software I had gotten as a gift from some credit card company back in the glory days. It contained state-specific forms where you could fill in the blanks. I printed up some before I left home and brought the software to install on his own computer to complete the rest.

That may have been the single smartest thing I did in the four years I was involved in his care.

These were basic forms and they looked like what they were: fill in the blanks, low-end legal documents. But they were properly signed, witnessed, and in one case also notarized. Over time I submitted them repeatedly to medical, legal, financial, government, and credit officials. I was the queen of the flying PDF. Not once did anybody's legal department say they were insufficient.

So don't let cost and/or fear of attorneys stand in the way of getting the paperwork you need.

In fact, at this point most of what you need can be done for free, working off various websites. And Nolo has a wide range of forms that will fill just about any legal need you might have, along with excellent free educational material on its website that explains all these matters in greater detail. www.nolo.com/

The simplest and most straightforward way to deal with all of this is probably to get the *WillMaker* software, which is bundled with any other forms you may need for Advance Directives, Powers of Attorney, and so on, and includes the proper forms for every state. This software worked through every stage of my brother's life and death in Illinois, and I just used a current version to update my own California legal paperwork.

There are plenty of free will-creating websites, though I would urge caution and can't specifically recommend any of them. If you choose to use one of these, look for forms that are state-specific. It's extremely important to do things exactly the way that South Dakota or New Mexico or Louisiana thinks you should. You don't want to end up in a jam with incorrect paperwork when you're also dealing with a medical crisis.

If it comes down to the wire, the reality is that just about anything is better than nothing. You may have to go to court to get a hastily-written, improperly witnessed document declared legal, but that's still better than having nothing at all. If it's all that you can manage, get a statement videotaped on your phone.

WILLS

Everybody should have a will, formally known as a Last Will and Testament, but a lot of folks are superstitious about the whole business.

If I make a will, I'll die.... It doesn't matter because everything will just go to my wife.... I don't want to think about it.... Let's do it tomorrow/next week/some other time.... What do I care?—I'll be dead anyway.

If any of these sound familiar, please try to adjust your thinking and bite down on this stick while we amputate your confusion and misinformation.

Wills are really, really, really important. The person whose worldly goods are at question may not be present when the will becomes a family reality, but he can count on being roundly cursed if there isn't one. Is that really how your brother wants to be remembered? As the dude who was too stubborn to write even the simplest will because he was so superstitious, and also so darned sure he'd live forever?

A will should be signed by the person making it in front of two witnesses who do not have any stake in the document itself as beneficiaries, executors, or other named relatives. If possible, it can't hurt to have it notarized, but this is not required in all states.

Anyone who believes that dealing with the legal and financial aftermath of a death (with or without a will) is easy has probably never done it. But even when there are complications, it's still easier with a Will because you will be working within predetermined legal rules for the appropriate jurisdiction.

LIVING TRUSTS

A trust is a legal document that gives one person the legal title to property for somebody else. A living trust is one that is created when you are alive. Living trusts generally come into play where significant assets and/or property are involved, and in those circumstances are designed to help avoid probate, reduce estate taxes, or handle the management of property.

This doesn't mean that you need to be rich to benefit from creating one, and while there are plenty of attorneys who would be happy to do this for you, there are also a lot of print and online resources if you want to do it yourself.

For more information about living trusts, see the excellent FAQs from Nolo at www.nolo.com/legal-encyclopedia/living-trust-faq-29036.html

DURABLE POWER OF ATTORNEY

This is what people generally mean when they say, very importantly, "I have power of attorney."

I used to say it all the time when I was handling my brother's affairs, and it opened a lot of doors, some of which I actually wish had stayed shut.

Durable Power of Attorney (POA) is the legal authorization to act on somebody's behalf for specific financial matters. It can be set up in all sorts of different ways, and just how specific those are depends on the individual and the situation.

Your sibling may want to severely limit financial authority, or to designate that major items may not be sold, or to impose a time limit. These are all valid options. Or you may be given *carte blanche* as I was, full authority to handle anything.

Normally at least one backup person will be listed on a POA. It's not a particularly wise idea to jointly designate people, however, especially if there are geographic considerations. Should you ever need to act quickly—and trust me, it happens—you don't want to be held up by arguments, or somebody being on vacation, or confusion over who can or can't do what.

Having power of attorney does *not* make you personally responsible for your sibling's debts or other financial obligations, only for trying to manage these to the best of your ability. With POA, you also have the authority to engage others to handle any or all of these matters. I hired a Realtor, real estate attorney, IRS enrolled agent, and several services on my brother's behalf, without a hitch.

No surprises, please. The person being given power of attorney needs to be aware that this is happening and to agree to accept the responsibility. Ideally it should be somebody trustworthy who understands basic financial matters and is capable of being sufficiently aggressive with bureaucrats and other functionaries.

In other words, somebody who knows how to get things done.

This may not be a spouse or child or even a relative. It certainly doesn't need to be a lawyer or accountant. Responsibility, availability, and willingness are the key factors.

WHY ALL THE DIFFERENT NAMES?

The legal paperwork that allows one person to make medical decisions on behalf of another has a whole lot of names, depending on where you live. So does the paperwork that lets you make those decisions in advance for yourself. These are often called a Durable Power of Attorney for Health Care and a Living Will. Some states combine them into one document and others require two. The simplest name is "Declaration" and the most complex, in Texas, "Directive to Physicians and Family or Surrogates."

The common nomenclature is **Advance Directives**, which usually covers both in the same document, and that's what we'll use here. But what it's called is a lot less important than its existence: a signed sheet of paper that says very clearly what your sibling wants in various medical circumstances, and who decides.

ADVANCE DIRECTIVES

Advance Directives designate who has responsibility to make medical decisions when the patient is not able to. This person is usually known as the Health Care Agent.

The Health Care Agent may authorize treatments, hire and fire doctors and other health care providers, and receive otherwise private medical information. HIPAA requirements have really tightened the dissemination of medical information, and without appropriate paperwork, you may find yourself flat out of luck when important decisions must be made.

All forms of Advance Directives provide an opportunity for an individual to make matters clear about just what kind of treatment she wants and what sort of life-sustaining equipment, measures, and philosophy should be used. She can also designate a preferred doctor, specify treatments and procedures she does (or doesn't) want, and give instructions for organ or body donation after death. She can specify what she does or doesn't want under certain circumstances. This may include a provision to continue pain relief and palliative care as needed, along with specification that she doesn't want a feeding tube, or additional surgery, or to be resuscitated.

Advance Directives can be modified or rescinded at any time.

People within the same family may have very different ideas on these subjects, so it's crucial to follow the patient's own wishes, as expressed in writing. Often these are based on observations of what parents or friends or other relatives did and didn't do: *I don't want to suffer like she did. … I won't give up like they did. … How did Aunt Elsie ever talk him into that surgery when he was already ninety-three?*

Options may be very specific or more general, and terminology may vary from one state to another. Whatever is specified, it's important to discuss and clarify everything with your sibling, at least to the extent that she is willing.

Advance Directives can be accessed through a Medic Alert service if your sibling wears a bracelet or dog tags.

Nolo is a superb resource for more comprehensive information on anything related to living wills and medical care directives. www.nolo.com/legal-encyclopedia/living-wills

DNR=DO NOT RESUSCITATE

A Do Not Resuscitate order is a very specific and

limited advance directive. It means that if your heart stops or you are not breathing, you don't want anybody to try to start up those processes again. The decision to use a DNR generally occurs in the final stages of a long and/or difficult illness, and it is never a decision made easily or casually.

A DNR order usually must also be signed by a treating physician. Copies should be on the refrigerator, bedside table, and in your sibling's (and your) purse or wallet.

At some point, your sister may decide that the next time she has a medical emergency that stops her heartbeat or respiration, she does not want to be resuscitated. That decision applies only to that one very specific situation. It does *not* mean that relatives, paramedics, and medical staff won't treat her for other medical emergencies or threats.

Her wishes may be ignored, however, if first responders don't see the DNR before they begin the work they are trained to start immediately, for instance when somebody collapses suddenly in a public setting.

In a hospital, a new internal DNR will be issued. This needs to be known to everybody involved in treatment, and should be clearly designated on the patient's chart. At home, any time paramedics are called for other reasons, they need to see the DNR before they see the patient, whose heart might be currently beating, but could stop in the course of treatment for whatever problem prompted the 911 call.

A MedicAlert bracelet or dog tag can and should note the DNR order. Paramedics check for that immediately.

If you have medical Power of Attorney, you can make the DNR decision with the doctor, though for obvious reasons it is preferable to have the document signed by the patient. Medical and residential facilities particularly prefer to have it signed by the patient. The assisted living facility or skilled nursing facility should have the DNR at the top of paperwork given to paramedics transporting a patient to the hospital, whether or not it seems relevant.

A DNR order can be revoked at any time.

POLST

As if all this weren't complicated enough, some states have yet another new form that you need to have if somebody is suffering from an advanced chronic or a terminal illness: the awkwardly-named POLST. This stands for Physician Orders for Life-Sustaining Treatment, and it typically lives on the refrigerator door or bedside table where paramedics will look for it first.

Like the DNR, this must be signed by a treating physician.

You may think this additional form isn't necessary if you already have a medical POA and Advance Directives and a DNR. But the problem is specificity. Your Advance Directives may say something about "quality of life" while your POLST specifies such particulars as no antibiotics, intubation, or feeding tube. All this is in medical terminology without any weasel words like "comfort." A copy of this belongs in the records of all your sibling's doctors and any hospital or facility where she is admitted or resides.

POLST supersedes a DNR, so that form is no longer necessary. It will be covered as part of the physician's specific instructions.

You can determine the status of POLST in your own state at www.polst.org.

In California, POLST is always on bright pink paper to make it obvious in a chart. So was my brother's DNR in his assisted living facility chart in Illinois. The point is to catch the eye, and hot pink will do that.

TO NOTARIZE OR NOT TO NOTARIZE?

Let's start with the basics. Exactly what is a notary public, besides one of the oddest job titles in modern life?

A notary public, also known simply as a notary, is an individual who is authorized to perform a number of legal-related functions without being an attorney. Training and licensing are both required. These requirements are state-specific, as are the situations in which simple witnesses are legally acceptable and in which notarization is required for Advance Directives. In general, financial POAs must be notarized.

Check with the source of your forms to see your state's requirements. You definitely want to get this one right.

It turns out that notaries can do all kinds of other things, but for the purposes of this discussion, the notary function in question is having legal documents witnessed. This must always be done in person, with the notary and the signatory in the same room at the same time.

The privacy of your documents is not at stake. The notary won't keep a copy, doesn't care what's in it, and won't be reading it. The notary's only job in this situation is to confirm your identity and to declare, with a big old notary public seal, that you are who you say you are. (By the time you reach this stage, you may already be wondering who you are.)

If you ask around, you can sometimes find a friend or relative who's a notary, perhaps in conjunction with work of some sort. Notaries generally charge a fee for their services, particularly if they need to come to you, as in a situation involving somebody who is housebound or in the hospital.

Many large offices have one, and large law offices almost certainly will.

I get documents notarized at my bank, and they do it for free.

GUARDIANSHIP AND CONSERVATORSHIP

Some medical situations develop gradually, such as a decline into dementia. Others appear in a moment, such as a stroke or aneurysm. If your sibling does not have paperwork in place designating who should make decisions for medical and/or financial matters, you may need to go to court to get appointed as guardian and/or conservator.

A guardianship gives you the power to take physical care of someone and authorizes decision-making in lieu of Advance Directives. A conservatorship permits you to manage financial affairs.

You will need a local attorney with experience in family law or estate planning to handle this for you and it won't be cheap. If you've got a situation requiring either, you are likely to need both and probably ought to do it all at once.

This only applies to the state where your sister is living.

If for some reason you need to relocate her to a different state, you may need to go through the whole process again, jumping through the same annoying and expensive set of hoops. Thirty-six states currently have enacted the Uniform Adult Guardianship and Protective Proceedings Jurisdiction Act. This does not change individual state laws, but establishes rules for communication between states to resolve jurisdictional issues.

WHERE ARE ALL THESE DOCUMENTS?

It doesn't do much good to have completed all this paperwork (at any point in history) if you don't have it available whenever and wherever it's needed. Copies are almost always acceptable and PDFs are easy to create at home and email anywhere. You can also store them on a phone or tablet. When I was dealing with new people on my brother's behalf, I was forever mailing and emailing POAs—but once people had that paperwork, I was usually able to deal indefinitely with whatever was at stake.

Make sure that all your sibling's doctors have Advance Directives on file, and provide them immediately to hospital personnel on admission or in the ER.

Apps have been created to store legal/medical documents and if you use a smartphone, it would probably be a good idea to get those apps and upload those documents. My Health Care Wishes, created by the American Bar Association's Commission on Law & Aging, is free and will let you immediately present documents by email or Bluetooth. www.americanbar.org/groups/law_aging/MyHealthCareWishes App.html

If you're already using a cloud-based storage system

like Dropbox, that will also work.

You may already have something on file with the doctor's office—the very doctor's office that just can't find it right now. Rather than trying to convince them they have it, you can whip out your phone or tablet and take care of it on the spot.

WHAT IF PEOPLE DISAGREE?

Even in public it's rare to find a family that agrees on everything, and behind the scenes it's pretty much impossible. When everybody is in total agreement about anything, I'm inclined to suspect that someone has sent in the clones.

We're all grownups now, more or less. The patterns of who agrees with whom on what are pretty well established and have been for decades. Even so, serious illness can bring out issues that have either never been discussed, or have surfaced briefly and then been swept into a dark corner.

Usually when there is an intense disagreement it's because the patient isn't able to currently participate in the decision-making. If she also didn't make her desires and intentions sufficiently clear before she became incapacitated, people may be insistent that they know what she would want.

Well, maybe. When this scenario has been studied, it seems that people tend to project their own ideas and beliefs so strongly that they often end up disregarding the actual wishes of the person who can't speak for herself right now.

Mediation of some sort can resolve these problems.

Start informally if you can, with a family member who gets along with everybody by virtue of being extremely diplomatic, unflinchingly neutral, or both. Step out of the way and let that person try to make the peace and bring people to a common ground.

A spiritual leader that everybody agrees on can come in handy here, but *only* if you all get along on religious matters, or the cleric in question is stunningly charismatic.

Professional mediation is available, and some municipalities have low-cost or free conflict resolution services for residents. Legal mediation will be a lot pricier, but is worth considering if money is not an issue and time is.

If the disagreements are intense enough and the players sufficiently strong-willed, you may need to go to court to get things resolved. Do try to avoid that. It's time and money spent in anger and counterproductive behaviors when everybody ought to be working together to create the best possible situation for your sibling.

Can't we all just get along? Not a bad mantra for family health crises.

ADDITIONAL INFORMATION

American Bar Association Commission on Law and Aging
www.americanbar.org/groups/law_aging.html

CaringInfo.com
www.caringinfo.org

Elder Decisions: Adult Family Conflict Resolution and Training
www.elderdecisions.com

Do-It-Yourself Legal Software and Forms from Nolo, Various titles
www.nolo.com/products

National Academy of Elder Law Attorneys (NAELA)
www.naela.org

POLST (Physician Orders for Life Sustaining Treatment)
www.polst.org/

• • • • •

Denis Clifford
Make Your Own Living Trust, 11th Edition
Nolo, 2013

Denis Clifford
Quick & Legal Will Book, 6th Edition
Nolo, 2011

Viki Kind
The Caregiver's Path to Compassionate Decision Making: Making Choices for Those Who Can't
Greenleaf Book Group, 2010

Rikk Larsen, Crystal Thorpe, and Blair Trippe
Mom Always Liked You Best: A Guide for Resolving Family Feuds, Inheritance Battles & Eldercare Crises
Agreement Resources, LLC, 2011

Nolo
Living Trust Maker Software, 3rd Edition
Nolo, 2010

Nolo
Quicken WillMaker Plus 2013
Nolo, 2013

Martin Shenkman
Estate Planning for People with a Chronic Condition or Disability
Demos Health, 2009

Kevin Urbatsch and Stephen Elias
Special Needs Trusts, 4th Edition
Nolo, 2011

Carol Elias Zolla and Liza Hanks
The Trustee's Legal Companion: A Step by Step Guide to Administering a Living Trust, 2nd Edition
Nolo, 2012

SECTION FOUR:

MONEY MATTERS

HEALTH CARE COSTS

Few things are as confusing, frightening, and expensive as medical care for serious illness in the 21st Century.

The fact that the baby boomers are moving into Medicare at the astonishing rate of 10,000 a day only compounds matters. And never mind the continual shape-shifting of the Affordable Care Act, known as Obamacare, and its various components. At the moment, American medical care remains a crapshoot in many ways, and you and your siblings are the dice.

You may get really lucky and have endless first-class medical treatment or you may have to fight for every X-ray and travel to India to find a kidney.

So you might as well accept up front that nothing is going to be cheap about this experience. And by the time you start worrying about money in a major medical emergency, you may already be a quarter-million in the hole.

For most of recent history, Americans tended to be only dimly aware of the costs of their health care.

For those with health insurance through an employer, very little choice was involved unless a spouse also had a job with health insurance or was entitled to some other form of medical care. You took what was offered, paid what was deducted from your paycheck, and assumed/hoped you would be covered if anything went seriously wrong.

Those without health insurance through employment did have choices, though they weren't terribly appealing. They might pay exorbitant COBRA costs after leaving a job, or find a no-frills policy with a huge deductible, or enroll in Medicaid if they were poor enough. Many simply went naked and prayed for good health.

Most people knew somebody who was insufficiently covered or totally uncovered when a serious illness or accident occurred. Community fundraisers and bankruptcy were the common outcomes in these situations, and it was not unusual for a family to lose everything fighting an illness which had a terrible conclusion anyway.

With the passage of the Affordable Care Act in 2010, much of that started to change.

By 2014, nobody could be denied for pre-existing conditions, there was no lifetime cap on covered expenses, kids could stay on their parents' policies until they were 26, Medicaid was expanded, certain preventive health measures become free, and eight million people were able to purchase insurance through the Healthcare.gov exchanges.

Make no mistake about it. This did not actually simplify anything. Insurance companies picked and chose the policies they would offer in particular states. Some states set up their own insurance exchanges and some declined to accept additional Medicaid coverage. Depending on location, somebody looking to purchase coverage might have dozens of options or only one.

The reality is that when you go to your doctor's office, there's an excellent chance that every single person in the waiting room has a different insurance policy with its own specific deductibles, co-pays and coverage limits.

MEANWHILE, BACK AT THE RANCH...

Health care costs had been skyrocketing without much media attention. My own individual private policy premiums doubled in the seven years before I went on Medicare, reaching an annual rate only slightly lower than what my parents paid for their first house.

Once it became clear that American health care was undergoing a sea change of tsunami proportions, however, investigative reporters started lifting various health care rocks. What they discovered was either everything you always suspected, or a terrible and unanticipated shock.

In either case, it wasn't pretty.

SOME BIG SURPRISES

The first rock rolled with a *Time* magazine Special Report in March 2013 by Steven Brill called "Bitter Pill" which was later expanded into a book, *America's Bitter Pill*. Brill confirmed something that many people had believed all along: Hospital charges bear no clear or even discernible relationship to what things actually cost. They are based instead on a secret price list known as a **chargemaster**. That chargemaster and its dazzlingly complex underpinnings represent the free enterprise system at its most fundamental: whatever the traffic will bear.

What's more, every hospital (or hospital chain) has its own different secret chargemaster. So two hospitals sitting side by side in a medical compound may have wildly different charges for essentially the same care. A joint replacement at one hospital might be billed at ten times more than at the hospital next door, with nobody the wiser except the insurance companies who get the bills. Private citizens are usually unaware of these price discrepancies, since patients go where the ambulance takes them or where the doctor sends them. People are a lot more likely to conduct consumer research on a new dishwasher than a new hip.

Anybody who's ever looked at a hospital bill will recall the obvious absurdities: the $45 aspirin, the $23 Band-Aid, the $19 sanitary napkin. But that's just the stuff that a lay person can recognize. When you start trying to figure out complex procedure names and lab tests and the additional charges related to those procedures, it is all but impossible to assess what's what, much less why.

Very few patients or insurers actually pay the full amount of any chargemaster item, however. That's because insurance companies all negotiate their own unpublicized payment schedules with hospitals and other health care providers.

For example, let's assume that the chargemaster lists Test 49-B for an inpatient at $100. Your insurance company may pay $57 for that test, while your next-door-neighbor's company pays $37 because they have more enrollees and thus more bargaining power. Medicare might assess it at $19.

If you're uninsured, however, you will be expected to pony up the full $100, unless you are prepared to pay cash on the spot for a price reduction. And if you are uninsured and don't pay anything, the hospital can write off the full $100 that it billed and dun you mercilessly.

That's one reason why Test 49-B is listed at $100. Another reason is that if a foreign billionaire shows up with a sackful of cash, he will probably pay the full amount without comment or concern.

It's like the rack rate for a hotel room posted inside the door, aimed at the wealthy traveler who might pay $400 for the same lumpy mattress and suspiciously-stained carpet that you thought was overpriced at $79.99. A seller who's willing to negotiate can ask for anything, after all, because somebody just might be willing to pay it.

Medicare reimbursements are much more uniform, though for some services they do vary based on regional rates and standards. Overall they are paid at lower rates than almost any other insurer. This does not mean, however, that the charges *submitted* to Medicare are lower, since the hospital is likely to bill the patient for amounts not covered by Medicare, co-pays and deductibles that may be the patient's responsibility without a Medicare Supplement or Medicare Advantage policy. Nor does it mean that the submitted charges are similar to those from other hospitals in the area.

Brill's report also focused on hospital administrative costs that went far beyond sending out those itemized, code-number-riddled bills. Top executives often receive annual compensation packages in the millions, while salaries dwindle sharply on their downward slide to the people actually providing patient care.

Once investigative reporters began looking at medical expenses, a lot of well-guarded medical financial doors began to crash open. *New York Times* reporter Elisabeth Rosenthal has produced a parade of well-researched articles examining medical costs, and other journalists have begun to follow suit. Rosenthal has looked at surgical costs, joint replacements, pharmaceutical expenses, devices, and more. What she discovered time after time was inconsistency, contradictions, and flat-out absurdity.

Rosenthal's work has spun off onto a very active Facebook group, Paying Till It Hurts.

HOW DO RATES GET SET?

So many medical charges are so outrageous that it's hard to single out any as particularly noteworthy, but my personal favorite is the way that Medicare determines the amounts that doctors are paid for performing various procedures.

Guess what? They ask the American Medical Association, the physicians' lobby. Then an AMA committee sends a questionnaire to doctors, asking them how long it takes to do the work they do and telling them why they're asking.

Yep, the fox handles security for the hen house.

To its credit, Medicare doesn't always accept those figures without question. Indeed, it often comes back with lower rates for less time. One can only hope that they completely discount figures from the numerous doctors who report that they routinely work more than 24 hours in any given day.

DOCTORS AND HEALTH CARE COSTS

If you ask your doctor what a procedure or test or

operation is going to cost, you will probably be told to check at the front desk or with the business office or to call your insurance company. Given the vast array of policies and coverage levels—remember that waiting room full of patients, all with different policies?—there probably isn't any good way to keep track.

A lot of doctors actually have no idea how things are billed and can't get straight answers themselves.

Some doctors, however, are much more aware. This is why, for instance, surgeons and other specialists like to have their own outpatient surgical and treatment centers. This allows them to bill directly for the many accoutrements of procedures that might otherwise be part of a hospital bill, such frills as anesthesia, operating room use, pre-op care, X-rays, and bandages. It also allows them to purchase expensive equipment and pass along those costs. Studies routinely show that physicians with their own facilities perform more procedures than their facility-free colleagues. One area that has been widely analyzed in this regard is colonoscopies, since they are now considered *de rigueur* for senior health care.

When the government recently began to release figures on how much physicians were paid annually by Medicare, some of the figures were truly shocking. A Florida ophthalmologist with good political connections got $21 million from Medicare in 2012, for example, after having been forced to repay $9 million for overbilling in 2007 and 2008. And it turned out that 2% of doctors accounted for about a quarter of the total payments, some $15 billion, with a quarter of the doctors overall receiving three-quarters of what gets shelled out.

These high payments don't necessary indicate malfeasance, malpractice, or fraud, however. It turned out that a single drug injected into the eye to treat macular degeneration in seniors was largely responsible for sky-high ophthalmology billings around the country.

There is also fraud, of course.

While examples of this are often shocking, they are also rare enough that I vividly recall a La Jolla ophthalmologist (ophthalmology again!) who was charged with Medicare fraud shortly after I moved to San Diego in the early 1990s. His case was complicated by the high regard in which he was held by both colleagues and patients, and his legal travails included revocation of his medical license and a criminal conviction. His website currently shows him licensed in Pennsylvania and practicing eye surgery internationally, apparent proof that there can be second acts for disgraced physicians.

ACCOUNTABLE CARE ORGANIZATIONS

One ongoing change in the health care industry is the rise of Accountable Care Organizations (ACOs) which are based on a concept of centralized care and billing, generally by a hospital or health care consortium. A patient's care is assumed by the ACO for a fixed fee no matter what and the emphasis is on efficiency and productivity.

Physicians in this model do not work for themselves or for their medical groups. They become salaried hospital employees, expected to produce at certain levels and to use the hospital's ancillary services and facilities for all care.

Right now nobody is entirely sure how this is going to work out, but in a world of uncertainty, this path is particularly appealing to young physicians. Stay tuned.

ARE HEALTH CARE COSTS NEGOTIABLE?

The answer here is Maybe.

You can certainly attempt to negotiate some charges by health care providers and facilities. I've done it myself, with limited success. The easiest type of bill to negotiate is from an individual provider who would rather have partial payment now than bill and harass somebody repeatedly before sending matters into collection later, with even less likelihood of ultimate payment.

Negotiation becomes progressively more difficult the larger the institution involved, however. A number of hospitals which once routinely extended charity care now expect some payment from nearly all patients and refuse to offer discounts to those whose income exceeds certain levels, generally a multiple of the national poverty level. Such facilities may offer payment plans without any overall fee reduction, or may make provisions for reductions in payment after putting applicants through various paperwork and income/resource verification hoops.

If you're faced with an impossible bill, you have nothing to lose by throwing yourself on the mercy of the billing individual or facility. You may not be able to work anything out, but the reality is that they aren't going to re-break your brother's leg or put your sister's appendix back in.

HEALTH CARE COSTS
AND PERSONAL CREDIT

Yes, this can screw up your sibling's personal credit.

If you owe money to a health care provider and don't pay promptly, whether through lack of funds or disputed charges, or even something as benign as not getting the proper bill, you have no way of knowing when that bill might go into collection. Nor do you control when the debt collection agency reports your fiscal tardiness to your credit bureau.

It's highly unusual to be aware what the bill is likely to be going into treatment, and absolutely impossible in the case of a medical emergency. This can move from an unexpected ambulance ride to three days in ICU faster than you can say "a hundred grand." Explanations of Benefits arrive in their own sweet time and are often impossible to understand.

What's more, once this lands on your credit report, it can be difficult to remove, even when you have paid off the obligation in full.

Be particularly wary of doctors or dentists who offer special health care credit cards and lines of credit. This concept arose for cosmetic surgery and other elective procedures not covered by health insurance, but now may be offered for care that is anything but optional. What's more, you can get this instant money right there in the doctor's office with some simple paperwork and a signature. A no-interest promotional period may seem appealing when dental pain is excruciating, but if the balance isn't paid in full within the allotted period, you can find yourself facing punitive late fees and retroactive interest rates as high as 30%.

ADDITIONAL INFORMATION

Steven Brill
America's Bitter Pill
Random House, 2014

Steven Brill
"Bitter Pill: How outrageous pricing and egregious profits are destroying our health care"
Time Magazine Special Report
March 4, 2013

Paying Till It Hurts Facebook Group
www.Facebook.com/groups/payingtillithurts

Elisabeth Rosenthal
"Paying Till It Hurts" (ongoing series)
The New York Times

PAYING FOR IT ALL

Medical bills are the single largest cause of bankruptcies in the United States, some 1.7 million of them in 2013. Be aware as you negotiate the maze of health care charges and payments that nothing is simple about any of these systems.

All of them include obstacles, limitations, and surprises.

SCROOGE McDUCK'S MONEY BAGS

Okay, I lied. If you pay for every penny of your own health care, there are no obstacles or limitations, though you are still likely to encounter surprises. These will most often come if you (or your bill-paying minions) look into the actual costs of things.

Yes, Virginia, there are people who pay cold hard cash at full price for their medical care and treatment in the United States. They may or may not be American citizens. Many wealthy foreigners come to this country because of the high quality medical care and treatment available here, and they are prepared to pay any price for that care. So are some Americans with extensive financial resources.

HEALTH INSURANCE

Prior to the passage of the Affordable Care Act in 2010, there was no guarantee that a person who wished to purchase health insurance could do so.

Most Americans were (and continue to be) covered through employer-sponsored health insurance. The employer determines the insurance company and terms of coverage, and the employee is obligated to use that policy under its specific terms, or to pay out of pocket for uncovered services and care.

Before the ACA, people who were self-employed, unemployed, or employed part time were on their own. Most insurance companies offered some individual policies, though the axiom was that you could usually get insurance only if you proved you didn't really need it.

Insurance companies could and did refuse to cover anybody for any reason, and could also cancel coverage pretty much at will. Most often this was because of pre-existing conditions, a minefield phrase that covers a world of medical territory. Available individual policies often carried huge deductibles and copays, a type of insurance known as catastrophic that is designed to lend a hand should you fall off a cliff or drop a refrigerator on your head.

COBRA policies for individuals entered the picture in 1986 with the Consolidated Omnibus Budget Reconciliation Act, providing the option to pay personally for the same coverage offered by a previous employer's health insurance policy after leaving a job. COBRA policies tend to be pricey and are generally good for no longer than eighteen months, the idea being that this will tide you over until you land a new job with health insurance benefits.

Everything began to change dramatically with the passage of the Affordable Care Act, also known as Obamacare. While the politics surrounding its passage and implementation have been dramatic and ceaseless, the reality is that millions of people have been able to procure insurance coverage through this legislation. Policies may be purchased either through state-established insurance exchanges or on the national www.Healthcare.gov website.

Policies are available at Platinum, Gold, Silver, and Bronze levels, with prices and benefits generally ranked according to how precious the metal may be. Fancy metal policies cost more but have better coverage, and subsidies based on income as related to the federal poverty level are available to any applicant who qualifies.

As time passes, it has become much easier to select a policy through the ACA.

The Affordable Care Act also established standards for what must be covered in every policy, including prescription drug coverage and various types of preventive care provided at no charge. The individual limits on annual and lifetime medical expenditures that were previously a staple of health insurance policies are gone.

Best of all for people who already have health issues, nobody can be denied coverage because of a pre-existing condition.

No matter what type of health insurance your sibling may be carrying, once you realize that you are in a situation where costs will be extensive, make at least a good-faith effort to clarify what is and isn't covered under the terms of that policy and at what payment rates. This includes charges and copays for specialists, drugs, and treatment facilities.

You'll want to know some of this to avoid sticker shock later, but it's also important if there is more than one policy involved because insurers are notorious for passing the buck—quite literally—in situations where there may be additional coverage of any sort.

Whatever the combination of insurance(s) may be, it should be clearly set out in all newly-completed medical paperwork and also in the Medical Notebook.

MEDICAID

Medicaid is a federal aid program for people with limited financial means who are unable to pay for health insurance. Like pretty much anything that originates in Washington, it is far more complicated than that.

Low means is one requirement for eligibility, but may not automatically qualify somebody. Medicaid is run at the state level, and states do not have to participate. Nor have they been required to accept additional Medicaid funding made available by the Affordable Care Act as part of its expansion of health insurance coverage.

And if that isn't enough to thoroughly befuddle you,

Medicaid also provides services by category, and these eligibility categories are extremely specific, though the only one you probably need right now is low-income senior. But we're not done yet. The interpretation of these eligibility categories varies from state to state, so that being eligible in one state may not transfer to another. Moving from California to Mississippi might be a very rude awakening.

Medicaid constitutes the lowest rung of the Affordable Care Act for applicants whose income falls below 133% of the federal poverty level.

One significant disadvantage to Medicaid is that not all doctors, hospitals, and other health care providers accept it. You or the patient's advocate may need to do some scrambling to find appropriate care and specialists.

This does not mean, however, that excellent coverage is not available, particularly in an emergency medical situation. I know personally of two uninsured people who received superb and successful cancer treatment through Medicaid. Both of these patients faced significant medical challenges, but both had also the advantage of informed and persistent advocates to negotiate the government maze to get the needed care.

If you need to get an uninsured sibling onto Medicaid in a hurry, try to find a social worker (perhaps associated with the hospital or medical practice) to help get you moving on the right track. This won't necessarily make anything easy. But it can at least save you the anxiety and pressure of charging blindfolded into arenas that seem expressly designed to make matters more complicated.

MEDICARE

Medicare has become such a thoroughly entrenched part of our national culture that it's hard to realize it didn't even exist until 1965, when it was enacted by Congress and signed by President Lyndon Johnson.

Medicare has served the Greatest Generation very well. They have generally received superb medical care that in some cases still continues as they move through their nineties and beyond.

Medicare does not only serve seniors, however. It is also a benefit attached to Social Security Disability payments for those younger than 65.

I used to fantasize about Medicare during the years when I was paying astronomical premiums for the only health insurance policy I could get as a self-employed individual with unremarkable pre-existing conditions. It couldn't come soon enough, and it would save me a fortune.

Now that I am enrolled in Medicare, I will confess I was surprised to learn that my fantasy object is far more complex than I had realized, something like a Disney prince who turns out also to have a doctorate in Medieval Studies and a sideline assisting Barbers Without Borders.

For starters, not everybody automatically gets Medicare. You need to have at least forty work credits over about ten years to even be eligible. If you don't qualify on your own work record, you may still be eligible through your spouse. You may also be able to buy in and pay a premium for coverage. (All of this is more complicated, of course.)

If you are 65 and eligible, Medicare Part A won't cost you a penny. If you are already receiving Social Security benefits, you will be automatically enrolled and your Medicare card will arrive one fine day a few months before your 65th birthday. If you aren't on Social Security, you can easily apply at www.medicare.gov/.

Alert readers will have already surmised that Part A generally doesn't exist without at least a Part B. In the case of Medicare, there are also Parts C and D, and every one of them is convoluted. I'll try to keep this as simple as possible.

Part A: Part A is hospitalization insurance. *Mandatory.*

Part B: Part B is medical insurance other than for hospitalization, including physicians, tests, treatments, and other medical charges. Part B carries a modest premium charge (deducted from Social Security if you receive that) and you need to actively opt out if you don't want it. *Optional but* *strongly recommended.*

    Part C: Part C is Medicare Advantage plans, which provide a combination of coverages. You enroll in a particular Advantage plan from a private insurer, which contracts with Medicare to provide your medical services for a flat monthly fee from the government. The insurer is billed directly for your Medicare A and B coverage. Some Advantage plans include Part D Prescription coverage as well. Advantage plans are HMO or PPO, and may have all kinds of different copays and deductibles. You pay the Medicare Advantage insurer directly. *Optional.*

    Part D: Part D is Prescription Drug coverage. This relatively new benefit began in 2006 and is also purchased separately from a private insurance company, either by itself or through a Part C Medicare Advantage plan. These plans have some standardization but vary significantly, and the best way to buy them is to work backwards from known prescription medication needs. You must enroll in these as soon as you are eligible, or you'll pay an eternal penalty for late enrollment. *Optional but strongly recommended.*

    Part PDQ: Medigap Insurance, aka Medicare Supplement plans, are purely private coverage, designed to pay for copays and deductibles not covered by Medicare. These policies also differ significantly and require research to assure adequate coverage. They do not include Part D Prescription Drug coverage. *Optional.*

    Medicare plans can also have complex interrelationships with other insurance.

    Research this carefully!

    I didn't, and when my brother's SSD-based Medicare coverage kicked in, I made some incorrect assumptions about how Medicare and his long-running, employer-issued coverage would interact. This provided to be an expensive mistake that I discovered only after some big bills for an overnight hospitalization came due.

    What should you do if somebody is still working and is covered (or has retired and is covered) by employer-issued health insurance? Start by checking with HR about coverage and then double-check by curling up with the Benefits booklet, that annually-issued doorstop that you normally don't even think about unless something has been denied.

Reminder to those whose eyes have glazed over: If you don't enroll in certain aspects of Medicare when you are first eligible to do so, you may need to pay a penalty forever after when you finally do sign up. However, you can take some small comfort in knowing there's a fairly brief grace period where you can correct mistakes made when you first enroll. In subsequent years, you can make changes to your Medicare coverage only during the winter Open Enrollment period.

If all of this seems hopelessly complicated and you aren't able to use the Medicare website to figure out what you need to know, look for one of the books on benefits. This is only slightly more expensive than banging your head on the wall, and has greater potential for providing necessary information.

MEDICAL CREDITORS

If you are being hounded by medical creditors, additional information about negotiation and creditor rights can be found in "The Paperwork Morass" chapter.

THROW A BENEFIT

There are times when you need a whole lot of money for a particular treatment or item, such as a wheelchair-accessible van for somebody whose mobility situation has just changed dramatically. If you are working with a sibling who is beloved in the community, you may be able to have some kind of benefit to raise money for such expenses.

This is a lot of work and requires time, talent, and energy that you probably don't have yourself just now. You need a really strong team to pull this off. The logistics alone are daunting, but if you have the right combination of need and enthusiastic volunteers, it can work.

You must, however, have the permission and full cooperation of your sibling for something of this magnitude, whether it's a glitzy gala or a spaghetti dinner in the church basement. Some people simply can't get past the idea of accepting such help, and if that's the case, you need to respect that refusal. This is not your illness.

FUNDRAISING BY LOCAL ORGANIZATIONS

You may find it easier to plug into existing community or church organizations if your sibling has a specific need. Service organizations exist (at least in theory) to help others and fundraising is one of their specialties.

Maybe the proceeds from the annual Kiwanis Pancake Breakfast can be earmarked for a motorized scooter, for example. Or maybe somebody in a particular club has an in with the auto agency that can come up with an appropriate (or at least adaptable) van at a really good price. This is where you can use all those contacts you made in the beginning of the SibCare journey.

Again, you need your sibling's agreement. If your brother is the kind of independent son of a gun who won't take a nickel if he finds it on the sidewalk, be sure he's on board before you start talking to the guys down at the VFW.

NOTIFY THE LOCAL MEDIA

People get sick all the time and it isn't exactly page one news. But there are times when you can take a particularly difficult situation and turn it into a newsworthy story.

Maybe there's been a denial of benefits to which you are certain your brother is clearly entitled. Or maybe some random doctor who happened to be in the ER but not in the appropriate network has sent a bill for $15K after a twenty-minute consultation. Perhaps the drug that is needed to hold Wellington's Wallop at bay costs $8,000 a pill and is about to double in price.

These are instances where you can sometimes interest a consumer reporter on the local TV network, or a reporter on the local newspaper, if you still have one. It's trickier to do this online, but social media may make it possible to call attention to the outrage in a way that will prove embarrassing to the party causing the trouble.

ADDITIONAL INFORMATION

Healthcare.gov
www.healthcare.gov/

My Medicare Matters
www.mymedicarematters.org/

The Official US Government Site for Medicare
www.medicare.gov/

US Department of Veterans Affairs
www.va.gov/
800. 827.1000

• • • • •

Lita Epstein
The Complete Idiot's Guide to Social Security & Medicare, 3rd Edition
ALPHA, 2010

Lita Epstein
The Pocket Idiot's Guide to Medicare Part D
ALPHA, 2009

Ronald A. Marks
Navigating the Social Security Disability Maze: Written Exclusively for Disability Applicants (Volume 1)
Golden Oriole Publishing, 2012

Dorothy Matthews Berman and Joseph Matthews
Social Security, Medicare and Government Pensions: Get the Most Out of Your Retirement & Medical Benefits, 18th Edition
Nolo, 2013

The Medical Bill Survival Guide: Easy, Effective Strategies for People Experiencing Financial Hardship
PlanetBiz Inc., 2010

Pat Palmer
The Medical Bill Survival Guide: What You Need to Know Before You Pay a Dime, Revised
Pat Palmer, 2012

SECTION FIVE:

MEDICAL CARE

DIFFERENT TYPES OF MEDICAL SITUATIONS

What you will need to do and how much assistance this will require are determined mostly by your sibling's medical condition, though other factors such as economics, geography, and personalities of the players may also come into play.

None of the following scenarios can be classified as "good," but some are far more pressing and problematic than others. There's also a lot of overlap. Odds are excellent that the situation you're confronting falls into one of these categories:
- Chronic or Long-Term
- Fast and Deadly
- Short-Term
- Intermittent
- Undiagnosed

CHRONIC AND LONG-TERM CONDITIONS

Chronic conditions generally come into play slowly over a long period of time and tend to be relatively stable, even as slow degeneration continues.

Long-term conditions are more likely to arrive quickly with little or no warning: heart attacks, major strokes, automobile accidents, falls resulting in serious fractures, brain injuries.

There's a certain amount of overlap between the categories, both in challenges and solutions. In both cases, the patient and SibCare team are signing on for the long haul, which may involve major lifestyle changes for everybody.

The word "chronic" derives from the Greek word for "time" and that says it all.

A chronic condition or illness becomes a part of your life, day in and day out. It may remain symptomatic at some manageable level for years, moving slowly, if at all. It may spend decades getting warmed up and diagnosed, particularly if its symptoms wax and wane. A lot of chronic conditions can and do plateau for years at a time, particularly if the patient is conscientious about following treatment regimens.

Many chronic conditions do signal a slow slide toward an unfortunate outcome, though emphasis is usually on the *slow*. You also generally have some treatment options along the way and the potential for a cure or treatment breakthrough in your lifetime. It never hurts to remind yourself at regular intervals of those white-jacketed scientists toiling in labs around the clock and around the world, seeking treatments and cures for pretty much everything. Your number could come up next time somebody strikes research gold.

Parkinson's disease is chronic. So are Multiple Sclerosis and lupus, since both may be held in check for long periods of time. Diabetes is a classic example, with the potential for lengthy plateaus if a patient is diligent about diet and ongoing treatment.

Diseases which were once squarely classifiable in the Fast and Deadly category can sometimes change their status, too. HIV/AIDS is now also a chronic disease that many people are able to live and work with for long periods.

The main distinction with long term situations is that they tend to follow a major medical event that makes abrupt and enormous changes in a person's life and lifestyle. The suddenness is a huge factor for everybody.

Major strokes are a good example, particularly those

where the patient eventually stabilizes at a level significantly below previous capabilities. Automobile or other accidents may result in lasting physical incapacities. Anything involving brain damage is likely to make permanent changes in your sibling's life—and by extension, everyone else's.

Some accidents start out relatively minor and grow more complicated over time, sometimes as a direct result of treatment. Attitude has a lot to do with accident recovery, but sometimes no matter how great your frame of mind, your body just doesn't get the message. After an initial period of treatment and adjustment and rehab, an accident victim probably won't get worse, but may not improve much, either. The danger becomes side-effects that can develop agendas of their own, such as slow-healing wounds in people with reduced sensation.

Unseen injuries can be just as devastating, if less physically dramatic. Brain injuries often leave no visible external signs to indicate that somebody has problems. Acquired brain injuries may arise from trauma or from strokes, seizures, tumors, or infections.

Traumatic brain injury (TBI) is currently the best-known type of brain injury, because of the tens of thousands of military personnel and civilian contractors who were too close to improvised explosive devices (IEDs) in the Middle East in recent wars. Symptoms of this battlefield TBI sometimes are delayed and may appear much later. This can complicate matters, particularly if the VA is involved.

Brain injuries of all sorts may manifest in a wide range of different (and changeable) symptoms, depending on the area of the brain affected and a person's overall health.

GEARING UP FOR THE LONG HAUL

When you're working with someone who has a chronic or long-term condition, things need to be set up to make the patient's independence as easy to maintain as possible for everybody involved.

This may mean physical modification of living quarters: installing wheelchair ramps and removing throw rugs and small tables that obstruct foot or wheelchair traffic patterns. Handrails in various locations are a huge help for those with balance or mobility problems. These are actually a pretty easy fix, can be relatively unobtrusive, and are a good idea for everybody on the sunset side of sixty.

At some point, hands-on caregiving with schedules and routines and maybe even employees is likely to become necessary for patients with advanced chronic or long-term conditions.

In general, chronic and long-term conditions are a one-way road with a downward slope, a slope that can turn much steeper with very little notice.

EXPECTATIONS AND TIMETABLES

It helps a family dealing with a chronic or long-term condition to understand reasonable expectations and timetables for likely changes. Since you're looking at a situation which will improve slowly if at all, this overview can help maintain equanimity over time. This is true even though there will always be somebody who isn't listening, refuses to hear, or stays stubbornly stuck on the wrong page.

Everybody who's involved with your sibling's care needs to be part of this information cycle and to address these issues:
- What is likely to happen next?
- How will this affect my sibling's life?
- How will this affect *my* life?
- How long will this stage last?
- Will new medications or treatment be required?
- What is likely to happen next?
- How will this affect my sibling's life?
- … and so on and so on and so on…

You may not yet have the fortitude to carry this sequence of events through to the end but you need to revisit it regularly. And it goes without saying that the patient should always be involved at a major level in this discussion unless there's a brain damage issue.

Fair is fair, and you'd expect the same courtesy.

FAST AND DEADLY

Fast and deadly illness strikes hard out of nowhere with one relentlessly focused goal: to wipe you out in the shortest possible period of time. It's the classic scene from the black-and-white movie where the patient says, "How long do I have, Doc?" and the kindly physician in the white coat replies, "Better get your affairs in order, son."

This type of illness can come on very dramatically.

Glioblastoma multiforme, the deadliest form of brain tumor, frequently announces itself with a grand mal seizure. Sepsis, a virulent form of infection often acquired during hospital stays, can explode into action and lay waste to a human body with terrifying speed. In the early years of the AIDS epidemic, a patient was often terminal by the time he was diagnosed, and getting to that stage didn't take long.

Some fast and deadly illnesses are actually slow and deadly, but provide no clues to their existence for years before they become noticeable. They may exhibit a variety of symptoms that seem unrelated and are not susceptible to customary treatments, while everyone despairs of ever getting an accurate diagnosis. Adding insult to grievous injury, malingering is sometimes suggested. Ovarian and pancreatic cancers are both extremely serious forms of the disease and notoriously difficult to diagnose.

THE MOMENT WHEN TIME STOPS

What many long-term and all fast-and-deadly situations share is that almost instantly everything changes forever.

One minute you're worrying about getting home in time to fix dinner. The next you are facing the strong possibility that somebody you love is going to die, and pretty darn quickly at that.

Medical decisions need to be made swiftly and acted upon without delay. Relatives and friends need to be informed and included if the patient is willing and held at bay if he isn't.

Denial is a luxury for which there simply isn't time. No time to dither, either, if that's your custom. All kinds of things need to be wrapped up ASAP.

PAPERWORK

You can't afford to let paperwork slide in either a long-term or fast-and-deadly situation, particularly medical-related paperwork that needs to be approved and signed by a patient who may be deteriorating rapidly. If you wait too long, you may need to get a conservatorship to oversee treatment.

You *really* need to have your sister sign Advance Directives designating who gets to make medical decisions when she can't and specifying the type of medical care she wants at the end of her life. You also need to press her to have some kind of will if she doesn't already.

This is not likely to be fun for anybody.

Plus this all has to happen at a time when nobody wants to do anything but pull the covers over their heads and sleep till a week from Tuesday. And never mind the screeching howls from every direction: *No! No! No!* countered by *Now! Now! Now!*

If everybody is grim and horrified and in shock from the rapid turn of events, you may be able to take care of all this legal paperwork during the initial collective numbness. Conversely, you may need to wait until that numbness passes, though this will eat up some valuable time.

During a period of familial paralysis, you may facilitate matters by making a point of doing the same paperwork for yourself and getting other family members to do so as well. You all ought to do that anyway. It may be your sister's illness right now, but anything can happen to any one of us, any time.

When somebody can no longer say what he wants, somebody else has to make that decision for him. If that person isn't clearly designated, the likelihood for disagreement among siblings and other family members is strong. It will also increase exponentially with each person you add to the decision-making equation. Eventually it will suck the oxygen out of everybody as the patient declines.

At a time when everybody ought to be pulling together and supporting one another, you're likely to end up in the middle of a knock-down, drag-out family fight, maybe even in court. Nobody outside of the litigation trade is ever enthusiastic about this kind of scenario.

If you're up against a patient who's resistant to signing (or even discussing) this legal paperwork, try playing the "go to court" card. Remind your brother that in addition to being expensive and inconvenient and having an uncertain outcome, going to court also takes his medical decision-making out of the family's hands altogether. Surely *that* isn't what your brother wants, is it? To have his care determined by some judge who doesn't even know him?

Do try to avoid all this. You haven't got time to appear on *The Jerry Springer Show.*

TOO MUCH, TOO SOON

You are likely to see your sibling's physical condition deteriorate in speedy and distressing ways. This kind of illness rarely looks like Ali McGraw in *Love Story.*

Everything happens in days, not months. Months, not years. Will an experimental treatment make a difference? Is there even time for one? How can it be only March? Christmas was about a year ago. What about hospice? And do you dare bring up memorial or funeral arrangements with the ailing sib?

Try to maintain your equanimity and as much as possible, take care of yourself. And if it's ever a question of spending time with your sibling or doing something that could wait, remember that right now almost everything else can wait.

SHORT-TERM MEDICAL SITUATIONS

As SibCare situations go, short-term is the pick of the litter.

By definition a short-term medical situation is ... short-term. It has a beginning, a middle and a probable, clearly-defined end. These boundaries may blur a bit now and then, but it's usually pretty straightforward.

Short-term situations which may require SibCare include most major surgical procedures—at least those unrelated to malignancy. This includes joint replacements, the bionic reinforcements that seemed deliciously exotic when Lee Majors and Lindsay Wagner had them on TV in the 80s, but have now become as commonplace as dandelions.

Currently they're mostly replacing hips and knees, but who knows what the future may bring? The human body has hundreds of joints, after all. We could be looking not too far down the road at bionic fingers and toes, and maybe even customized joint replacements like the Super-Supple Yoga Goddess hip.

Survivors of heart attacks and minor strokes may need and want some short-term assistance as well. This works particularly well when the patient has already made a significant recovery and is committed to whatever lifestyle changes have been recommended to prevent a recurrence. This kind of SibCare may amount to little more than transportation to a few doctor appointments along with plenty of moral support and attaboys.

The object here is for everyone to get back as quickly as possible to their regularly scheduled lives. You want to help your sibling regain independence swiftly and painlessly in the new normal for her current medical condition. Environmental modifications such as wheelchair ramps, handrails, and scooping up the throw rugs may be necessary either for the short or the long term.

Scheduling is important in short-term situations, particularly where rehab or other therapy continues, but it isn't the complex spider web that may be necessary in more lengthy or intense medical situations.

You'll still want to be sure the patient's legal paperwork is in order, but it's a lot easier to do this when there's less obvious and immediate danger. You can make light of the process and maybe all the sibs can do it together, except for that smug sister whose regularly-updated will has been on file with her attorney since 1974.

Do whatever it takes to get your sibling to make Advance Directives. Hospitals and physicians may aid you by pushing this as well.

Surgery always carries risks, anesthesia multiplies those risks, and not every outcome is ideal. Much surgery is performed at outpatient surgery centers, where your sibling will be released within hours. Back home, everyone needs to stay particularly alert, just because. Going to the hospital is scary on many levels, including bad reactions to who-knows-what and those hideous hospital-borne infections.

You might try to keep the discussion on the lighter side by referencing Woody Allen in *Sleeper,* where he went into the hospital for something minor and woke up 200 years later. Then after the surgery, maybe you can watch *Sleeper* together. Remember the scene where the 200-year-old Volkswagen starts right up?

INTERMITTENT SITUATIONS

Many medical problems can go for relatively long periods between flare-ups or exacerbations or relapses, whatever a particular disease calls it when bad symptoms suddenly appear front and center, clamoring for attention. In many of these cases, your sibling's need for outside help is likely to be intermittent, and may even provide some warning.

It's also possible that your sib's problem is one which will require treatment at regular intervals over a prolonged period of time, such as chemotherapy.

In this kind of situation, once you get a routine of some sort set up—automatic scheduling of drivers, for instance—then it's just a matter of swinging back into action as the need arises. Figure out the drill by trial and error, and then fall back on those procedures as you need to.

Or, as they say in the medical world, "prn."

If your sibling's treatment schedule is relatively long-term and rigid, such as a lot of oncology regimens, then you can form a reasonably clear timetable and can plan ahead. This allows for the luxury of scheduled time off work or using bargain airfares.

But always build in flexibility as a component of intermittent situations. Because the flip side of this tidy scheduling is that when somebody is seriously ill, there's always a chance of a sudden change. And that change could be almost anything.

WHY IS THIS HAPPENING?

When a boomer who's been smoking three packs a day since freshman year in high school gets lung cancer, nobody asks why. Sometimes it's all too obvious how a person went from Lifestyle A to Diagnosis B.

Most causal relationships leading up to illness or affliction aren't quite that straightforward, but when something bad happens, we want to know why.

When the answer to "Why?" is "Nobody knows," it's called *unknown etiology* and it can be a real bitch. How can you make sure something doesn't happen again when you don't even know why it happened the first time?

However, it's important to remember that not knowing the precise cause of something doesn't mean it can't be treated, and treated successfully. Usually there isn't much point in tying yourself in knots trying to figure out just why this is happening. You have other things to take care of right now, such as treating the affliction or building wheelchair ramps, or trying to recruit more help to care for your sib when you go home next Thursday.

For the record, most active smokers diagnosed with lung cancer *do* quit smoking. And some people who have never smoked get lung cancer.

WHAT IF YOU CAN'T GET A DIAGNOSIS?

One of the most frustrating situations anyone can face is being very ill—with symptoms that are absolutely real and quite terrible—and not knowing what you have.

Medical science has difficulty diagnosing quite a few ailments, though certainly there are fewer of these now than, say, a hundred years ago. At the same time, there are thousands more specific diagnoses than there used to be. Mostly this has to with differentiating among similar diseases once lumped together. "Palsy" or "consumption" or "insanity" were old-time diagnoses that covered a lot of territory.

These days we tend to believe that if you perform enough testing you will eventually figure out what's wrong. Devotees of the recent medical TV series *House, M.D.* will recognize this as the period when vasculitis is ruled out.

While this testing is going on, of course, what are known as the "presenting symptoms" are still presenting and also presumably being treated. So the good news is that when you do finally get a diagnosis you'll most likely already be undergoing appropriate treatment.

But the nightmare while you wait for a diagnosis is the uncertainty. If medical science can't even figure out what's wrong with you, how can you possibly get better? There's no ambiguity comparable to having major physical problems with no idea what is happening or why.

Nor does it necessarily do you any good to be privileged or educated.

A couple of decades ago the 52-year-old husband of a college friend became extremely ill. Nobody could figure out what was wrong with him, and a lot of very competent people gave it a really good shot, at least in part because he was a wonderful guy. He was also a graduate of Harvard Medical School and spent a month as an inpatient at the Mayo Clinic in search of a diagnosis. If ever somebody got the platinum treatment from the medical profession, he was the one.

Even so, by the time he finally was diagnosed with liver

cancer, he was only a few weeks from death.

This doesn't mean that your undiagnosed sibling is going to die. It's a reminder that being unable to identify the nature of your medical enemy doesn't necessarily indicate a problem with your medical team.

You have to hope and assume that the attempts that team is making to treat your brother's symptoms will at least offer him some relief, even if nobody knows what they are symptoms of. This happens a lot more frequently than anybody is willing to admit.

Sorry. Nobody said this would all be pretty.

ADDITIONAL INFORMATION

Partnership to Fight Chronic Disease
www.fightchronicdisease.org/

• • • • •

Laurie Edwards
In the Kingdom of the Sick: A Social History of Chronic Illness in America
Walker & Co., 2013

Robert A. Norman and Linda Ruescher
100 Questions & Answers About Chronic Illness
Jones and Bartlett, 2011

Joy Selak and Steve Overman
You Don't Look Sick! Living Well With Chronic Invisible Illness
Demos Health, 2012

DOCTORS IN 21ST CENTURY AMERICA:

MARCUS WELBY HAS LEFT THE BUILDING

My father was a surgeon who operated most weekday mornings, starting his first case at 7:30 AM because he didn't want to wait for an operating room. After surgery, he made hospital rounds to visit all his currently-admitted patients, who generally went home after about a week. On days when he didn't operate, he'd make morning rounds before his afternoon and/or evening office hours. On weekends he sometimes made rounds in a sports shirt—but make rounds he did.

His flat fees included all pre-op, post-op, and hospital visits and were, as I think about it now, quite reasonable. An appendectomy cost $600 when I was in high school.

Back then, if you were in the hospital for something other than surgery or childbirth—a heart attack, perhaps, or a bleeding ulcer—your family physician saw you before, during and after that hospitalization. If you came into the Emergency Room, the ER called your family doctor.

Who showed up.

Interns and residents worked ridiculously long hours to coordinate most of your hospital care while your doctor was elsewhere. That care was provided by registered nurses in starched white uniforms, white nylons, and ugly white shoes with corrugated rubber soles. Their crisp white caps were unique to their various alma maters and occasionally quite fanciful.

About all that remains today of that medical model is the overworked residents.

WHO *ARE* ALL THOSE DOCTORS?

When my sister and I first got actively involved in our brother's medical affairs, we were surprised to learn just how compartmentalized medical care had become. Physicians have specialties and sub-specialties that not only didn't exist a generation ago, but wouldn't even have been imagined then. I recently read a book by a doctor who specializes in surgery for cancer of the endocrine glands and I had to look up exactly what that meant.

In the course of a single medical adventure, your family may have reason to consult several specialists, a kind of forced march through body parts and medical waiting rooms. In the year following his first stroke, my brother was treated by four primary care physicians, four neurologists (two of whom were epileptologists), a neuropsychologist, two rehabilitation specialists, a rheumatologist, a psychiatrist (briefly and against his will) and maybe a witch doctor or two. The multiples are because he lived in three different geographic areas through that year, but that's still half a dozen specialties.

Except for the rehab docs, that did not include the physicians he saw while hospitalized on four separate occasions.

Doctors inside the hospital are another subspecies altogether.

If you come into the hospital through the Emergency Room, the doctor you see will be involved in your care only until you are discharged or admitted. **Emergency room specialists** do just that: treat emergencies as they come through the door. Then they go home and you only see them again if you become an ER regular.

The ER doc will notify and consult with **a relevant specialist** and/or **your primary care physician,** particularly if what seems to ail you has a history that could be useful and you are being admitted. It's entirely possible that you won't see your regular doctor at all while you're in the hospital, but you may see one or more hospitalists, depending on what's wrong with you.

Hospitalists are doctors who treat you only while

you are a patient in the hospital. Hospitalists often have medical specialties, so the person who's seeing you may also have an outside practice, particularly if he's a specialist of some sort, such as a urologist or a neurologist.

Should you spend time in Intensive Care, your hospitalist will be an **intensivist.**

When you are discharged, your regular team of physicians takes over again, at least in theory. If you don't have a regular team of physicians, or are the kind of person who never goes to the doctor at all, this is a particularly weak link in the care cycle. At this point somebody new needs to be recruited in a hurry, or the ball gets dropped.

If things have gone well with that hospitalist, and she also has a private practice, you may already consider this problem solved. If not, make sure that you get some recommendations from the hospital before discharge. A choice, if at all possible.

As quickly as hospitals like to get people in and out, they do try to be responsible about discharging seriously ill people into somebody's care. Also they are now penalized by Medicare, the health care world's five-hundred-pound gorilla, if they send too many people home early and then have to re-hospitalize them. Penalized financially.

AREN'T THEY AWFULLY YOUNG?

It's been a staple of aging comedians since the audience draped itself around the Roman baths in togas: references to the ridiculously young doctor who still has pimples and sleeps in footie pajamas. Doogie Howser, though not necessarily cute. And yes, there are quite a lot of young doctors these days.

I've grown quite comfortable with younger doctors. They represent the best and brightest of some very talented and intelligent peer groups, they generally know a lot about their specialties, and you can assume that their medical information has to be relatively current simply because they haven't been accumulating it all that long.

In fact, there are some instances where you *want* to

have a young doctor, where there may not even be a choice.

Perhaps the most obvious is robotic surgery, used in some of the most delicate surgical procedures and the almost-exclusive province of the young. Why? Because these kids grew up with computers and gaming. They are far more comfortable with the remote manipulation of surgical tools than those old folks who learned to perform surgery with scalpels and retractors.

FOREIGN DOCTORS

Thousands of foreign-trained immigrant doctors living in the United States would love to be licensed to practice medicine here. Many of these are people with exceptional training who were licensed and highly regarded in their countries of origin, and who now work at significantly lesser jobs in the medical sector while they traverse the torturous path to licensing.

That path is an expensive and lengthy obstacle course that includes all manner of requirements and one huge bottleneck: residency. The limited funding for residencies, essential for virtually all specialties, comes mostly from Medicare (who knew?) and has been frozen by Congress since 1997. As it is, there aren't enough residency slots to accommodate all the US citizens who graduate from US medical schools, not to mention the US citizens who studied medicine abroad because they couldn't get into med school at home.

Immigrant doctors have been arriving on these shores since shortly after the Pilgrims disembarked at Plymouth Rock. Back in the early 1960s, my father's hospital employed a group of interns who were post-revolution refugees from Cuba. I met many of these doctors while working on a special project at the hospital one summer and while I wasn't in any position to judge their medical expertise, I do recall that all of them were quite charming and one had been the Cuban Minister of Health.

Not everybody who wants a medical license should be

able to get one, of course. This is why standards exist. However, expediting some of the processes for residency and the licensing of qualified foreign nationals to practice medicine would seem to be an important and logical component of an expanding demand for medical care. How the medical community will respond to this increased need remains to be seen.

BOARD CERTIFICATION

Once a physician is licensed, that isn't the end of it. Increasingly doctors are Board certified in their specialties, and some hospitals and medical groups *require* certification.

A physician becomes board certified by passing a specific examination in the field of specialty. This may include some kind of practical exam as well as the traditional written test, and certification is overseen in the US by the following entities:

- The American Board of Medical Specialties and the American Medical Association.
- The American Osteopathic Association Bureau of Osteopathic Specialists and the American Osteopathic Association.
- The American Board of Physician Specialties and the American Association of Physician Specialists.

Does this mean that Board certified doctors are better than those who aren't certified? It may. It does definitely means that at some point, the doctor demonstrated proficiency and knowledge of the core information required for a specialty in a particular field.

SECOND OPINIONS

Doctors do not agree on everything and they don't all know the same stuff.

Second opinions are important—sometimes at the diagnosis stage, sometimes as treatment options are considered, and sometimes for both. There may not be a lot of time for this in the case of a fast-moving cancer or a complicated fracture requiring surgery, but you should always keep it in mind.

When you are facing major medical treatment of any kind, many insurance companies both encourage and require second opinions. They can also be worth every penny even if you have to pay for them yourself.

It's easier to shop around if you're in a good-sized metropolitan area, but worth investigating alternatives no matter where you live. If you live smack in the middle of nowhere, consider a road trip.

Ideally, you want your sibling's treatment handled by people who do this kind of work a lot. Surgery, for example, has grown extremely specialized, with people limiting their practices to operations on a single organ you may never have heard of before. You're likely to do better with a surgeon who handles two hundred similar cases a year rather than four. Similarly, an oncologist at a teaching hospital may be aware of new possibilities that haven't yet reached the medical personnel in your town. These situations are even more urgent if you are fighting a difficult or obscure form of a very nasty disease.

Second opinions are not just for life-threatening situations, however. Trust your gut. If you have an uneasy feeling that maybe the current medical team doesn't quite know what it's doing, or if things have been muddling along for quite some time without a hint of progress, you absolutely need another take on the situation. Even if your sister adores her primary care physician.

Remind her that just because you seek a second opinion, you don't have to take it. It may simply confirm what her doctor has been saying, reassuring in its own right.

This is not an insult to the doctor. If a doctor is bothered that you want another health professional's assessment, that's a red flag all by itself. The doctor's job is to concentrate on the patient's well-being, not his own ego.

THE GOD COMPLEX

People on the top tiers of various professions are often

pretty full of themselves, generally with good reason. It isn't easy getting to the top of any field. But medicine's top tier sometimes exhibits an attitude so institutionalized that it has a name: the God Complex.

Most people who have regular medical checkups or treatment will recognize this character instantly: omnipotent and omniscient because he is the doctor and you are not, and also because he's been doing this for many, many years.

The God Complex, as is the case with many stereotypes, is based on a pretty firm foundation. A physician does possess the power to save lives, to bring forth life through childbirth, and to see it through to its inevitable conclusion on a patient's deathbed. All intermediate steps are covered as well.

In some ways a physician with a God Complex is similar to the egomaniacal actor who spent too much time reading his own great reviews and boffo box office figures and now wants to control the entire film industry and a couple of small countries.

In other ways the situation is entirely distinct, and not just because actors can't write their own prescriptions, much as they might like to.

A doctor with a God Complex running at full speed expects obedience from patients and support staff alike and is not likely to tolerate any form of dissent. He burns through underlings, is usually uninterested in ideas presented by others, and may not listen very carefully. On the playground he'd be considered a bully, though odds are good that back when he *was* on the playground, he was the one who was being beaten up.

Unless there is some really compelling reason to tolerate such behavior, I recommend leaving these doctors to their own petty fiefdoms and seeking out somebody else.

WHAT IF THE DOCTOR IS WRONG?

Do doctors make mistakes? Of course they do.

Do doctors know that they make mistakes? Of course they do.

Do they admit that they make mistakes?

Well, that one's kind of tricky and depends on a lot of variables, some of which are likely to be legal in this litigation-frenzied era. But when doctors screw up significantly and are aware of it—two items that are not automatically linked—the awareness is likely to stay with them forever.

Some mistakes are simple and straightforward. If an orthopedic surgeon cuts off the wrong leg, the evidence is difficult to miss. It's hopping into the courtroom.

Most physician errors are a lot more subtle and are likely to involve a missed or delayed diagnosis. That in turn might come from treating a complaint that is generally outside the physician's area of expertise.

Some errors also arise through the very nature of the specialty-splintered profession and its relationship to multiple health insurance companies. A doctor may be seeing a patient with problems that aren't in her treatment comfort zone, and if the patient's insurance company makes it difficult to consult a specialist, that further complicates matters. Meanwhile, a symptom may be missed or underestimated, so a possible field of diagnostic exploration is eliminated.

Once medication enters the picture, you also have the potential for not helping the original problem or making matters worse through side effects or interactions with other necessary medications.

All of this gets dangerous when the wrong diagnosis actually harms the patient. This is the juncture in *House, M.D.* when the patient turns turquoise or starts spewing blood from miscellaneous orifices. In real life it's generally not so desperate or dramatic, but nobody really likes to admit they are wrong and doctors are not an exception.

Try not to worry too much about these issues, but if you're troubled for specific reasons or if your research suggests your sibling's medical train is on the wrong track, speak up.

HOW CAN YOU FIND OUT
ABOUT DOCTORS?

Physicians are licensed by the states they practice in, and licensing is no simple matter. Once that license is granted, however, keeping it updated and renewed is relatively simple.

It's hard to know who to believe about doctors. The average person is often clueless and asking around doesn't always help. Your friends may like their primary care physician because he reminds them of their doctor back in Dallas, or because he oversaw the successful treatment of a difficult problem, or because he is personable, or because he looks like George Clooney. That doctor may be somebody who was assigned under terms of their health insurance. Or he may be a doddering old fool with 1950s medical charm, which is not much of an asset in the technological arenas of the 21st Century.

You have no way of knowing.

There is at least one relatively objective measure, however: HealthGrades.com. You can plug in a doctor's name here and see how other people have rated her on a range of factors, based on a series of specific questions about their interactions with the doctor. You can also learn where she was trained and what additional certification she may have in her specialty. The site will also let you know if the doctor has a history of malpractice claims, sanctions, or board actions on record.

HealthGrades ratings beat random recommendations because they are a bit more objective and have a broader base of reporters. This site is also an excellent way to compare qualifications of specialists if you need one. www.healthgrades.com

ARE DOCTORS INDISPENSIBLE?

It depends on who you ask, and I think we all have a pretty good idea what the response is from the AMA.

Some doctors are throwing up their hands and saying

the hell with it, that Obamacare is ruining everything (which hasn't happened yet) and Medicare doesn't pay them enough (which is true) and that it just isn't worth messing with any of it. More doctors are opting out of taking Medicare patients than ever before, though it's still a very small percentage.

This reminds me a bit of when HMOs first swept through the California medical industry a couple of decades ago and some doctors got all huffy and moved to states like Kentucky where they could practice the way they wanted with nobody telling them what to do. It made a little jiggle in local medical service and then nobody ever mentioned it again.

I am certainly not advocating getting rid of doctors, who include a lot of wonderful, dedicated, informed, and caring people—along with a few misfits, incompetents and cranks, just like any other field.

But I admit to a small amount of pleasure at watching the medical profession play Ignore-it-and-then-Scramble yet again.

ALTERNATIVES TO DOCTORS

I believe that the use of other types of medical practitioners to provide some of the care currently the province of doctors is all but inevitable.

Some doctors get annoyed by this, but the reality is that not everything that doctors do needs to be done by doctors, and there are only 24 hours in a day. If you are making your goal to provide the best possible medical care to the greatest number of people—as we all hope our doctors are—it makes sense to use your resources wisely.

Physician assistants, nurse practitioners, and **midwives** are trained and licensed to provide specifically enumerated medical tasks. Most of the time they are very good at what they do, and are often more personable than the physicians they work with.

According to the American Association of Physician Assistants: "PAs perform physical examinations, diagnose and treat illnesses, order and interpret lab tests, perform procedures, assist in surgery, provide patient education and counseling and make rounds in hospitals and nursing homes." They can also prescribe medications.

In short, they can do pretty much the same thing that doctors do, working as part of a team with a licensed physician.

Physician assistants have at least two years of college, go through rigorous and competitive training, and are licensed by their state. They can be particularly useful in rural or isolated areas not served directly by licensed physicians and are sometimes supervised at a distance by electronic communication. There are currently about 90,000 physician assistants in the US, a bit more than one for every ten licensed physicians.

Nurse-practitioners are registered nurses with advanced degrees. Nationally certified and licensed by their states, they perform most of the same functions that physician assistants do, including writing prescriptions. Physician assistants and nurse-practitioners are most commonly found in family practice or women's health settings.

Both of these occupations are rank newcomers compared to midwives, who have been around about as long as women have been having babies.

THE ART OF ELECTRONIC DIAGNOSIS

A dandy new development on the computer front is also likely to make older doctors a little uncomfortable, particularly if they have never taken very well to the computer age. But it will be greeted with enthusiasm by younger, more tech-savvy doctors as the baby boomer docs continue to retire.

Remember that IBM computer that was programmed to play *Jeopardy!* against mega-champions? It did quite well at that, thank you very much. And now that it's whupped mankind's ass in the game show realm, it's being taught to assist with medical diagnosis.

Yes. A computer will help your doctor figure out what's wrong with you. Far from where someone is being examined in a medical professional's office, the computer will be able to assess the patient's symptoms and offer possible diagnoses and treatments in simple checklist form. These suggestions will be based on extensive data and as more and more data is accumulated and added, the system is expected to get even better.

The idea, of course, is both to streamline the diagnostic process and to make sure that less obvious diagnoses which might arise from similar symptoms are also explored. Doctors aren't likely to seek a more esoteric explanation for a medical problem when a perfectly obvious and relatively familiar one is sitting right in front of them. Jerome Groopman spends a lot of time on the diagnostic process in his fascinating book, *How Doctors Think.* So does Lisa Sanders, who served as medical consultant on *House, M.D.,* in *Every Patient Tells a Story.*

The medical world, however, is not populated by folks like Dr. House, with one patient, a staff of highly trained assistants and a mission to determine which exotic affliction has downed the patient of the week. It's full of men and women who have large caseloads, families, professional obligations, payrolls to meet, and a limited number of hours in the day.

ARE THERE GOING TO BE ENOUGH DOCTORS?

Half of the 830,000 licensed doctors in the United States in 2012 were over the age of fifty. That includes the entire baby boomer generation.

It would be nice to report that as the boomers retire they are being replaced by increased numbers of enthusiastic young physicians entering the field as an avocation to care for the ill with little consideration of financial reward. It would also be a lie.

Today's brand new physician is hauling around up to a quarter million dollars in student debt, which makes that family practice in the small Southern town a lot less appealing than the allergy specialty in Atlanta.

Today's brand new physician is also the product of the

most rigorous academic standards ever applied to aspiring doctors. Back in the Depression when my father went to medical school after an extremely lackluster undergraduate career, all you really needed to get in was some kind of college diploma and a fistful of money. Boy, has *that* changed.

A whole lot more people want to go to medical school than ever get in today, and the winnowing process generally starts with a couple of really tough undergraduate science courses. Students who start out as pre-med begin to drop by the wayside as coursework becomes more strenuous and competing GPAs soar.

By the time the top survivors in the US reached the med school application process in 2012, they had self-selected down to a very modest 45,266 applicants throughout the entire country. (For purposes of perspective, there were twice as many applicants to the UCLA undergraduate program the same year.) 43% of those applicants, or 19,517, were accepted to medical school.

Obamacare has made basic preventive medical care available to large numbers of people who haven't had that opportunity before. At the moment, there are less than three doctors per thousand people in the United States, and that includes quite a few specialists. I'd like to report that the medical profession recognized this future development immediately (more customers!) and created a collective business plan to expand its numbers significantly to meet the challenge. That would also be a lie.

There is, however, one silver lining to this looming doctor crunch.

Back in 1970 when I graduated from college, only 7.6% of the doctors in the entire country were women. For the next fifteen years or so, whenever I needed a doctor and had no trusted local referral source, I chose new doctors purely by gender. My reasoning was simple: To become physicians at all, these women had to be so much better than the male competition that they probably also practiced pretty good medicine. In most cases, that proved correct.

We've come a long way. Today a third of the licensed

physicians in the United States are women, as are nearly half the students entering medical school.

ADDITIONAL INFORMATION

American Medical Association (AMA)
www.ama-assn.org/ama

HealthGrades: Find a Doctor/Doctor Reviews/Hospital Ratings
www.healthgrades.com/

• • • • •

Otis Webb Brawley with Paul Goldberg
How We Do Harm: A Doctor Breaks Ranks about Being Sick in America
St. Martin's Press, 2012

Joe Graedon and Teresa Graedon
Top Screwups Doctors Make and How to Avoid Them
Three Rivers Press, 2012

Jerome Groopman
How Doctors Think
Mariner Books, 2008

Jerome Groopman and Pamela Hartzband
Your Medical Mind: How to Decide What is Right for You
Penguin, 2012 reprint

John King and Cynthia R. King
100 Questions & Answers About Communicating with Your Healthcare Provider
Jones and Bartlett, 2009

Andy Kessler
The End of Medicine: How Silicon Valley (and Naked Mice) Will Reboot Your Doctor
HarperBusiness, 2007

Robert Klitzman
When Doctors Become Patients
Oxford University Press, 2008

Leana Wen and Joshua Koslowsky
When Doctors Don't Listen: How to Avoid Misdiagnoses and Unnecessary Tests
Thomas Dunne Books, 2013

HOSPITAL WORLD:
MYTH VS. REALITY

Not all that long ago, when somebody was admitted to the hospital with a serious medical problem, everybody heaved a sigh of relief. Things would be better now. The patient would be cared for by skilled medical staff and sent home to recuperate only when she was ready. Everybody would live happily ever after.

The camera is still aiming at the same outcome, but much about that picture has a very different focus now.

For one thing, when somebody is admitted to the hospital today, a major concern is getting the patient back out alive.

Some of the nastiest infections known to humanity hover around hospitals, hoping to swoop in and take over the bodies of patients whose health is already severely compromised. This seems counterintuitive in a world exploding with medical research, new treatment possibilities, and advances being announced on dozens of medical fronts daily, but it's a cold hard fact.

At the same time, only the sickest of the sick are admitted at all, and they are generally wheeled back out the door at the earliest possible opportunity, sometimes into a rehab facility to continue recovery but more often right back home. When they started doing drive-by mastectomies a few years back, I realized the slope wasn't just slippery anymore.

It had turned into a multistory waterslide worthy of a Las Vegas hotel.

INTRODUCING THE CHECKLIST

As anyone who has tried to change a well-entrenched culture will attest, the toughest sentence in the language to combat is: "We've always done it this way."

Dr. Peter Provonost at Johns Hopkins Hospital decided that wasn't a good enough answer back in 2000 and set about reducing infections in one very specific area of care: central line catheters. Central line catheters are inserted through blood vessels near the heart of someone who is already severely ill, to allow for the efficient administration of fluids, medications and nutrients.

Provonost concentrated on breaking the situation down to its simplest elements, those common to all patients using this equipment. He chose the aviation industry as a model, noting that checklists used by pilots for nearly every aspect of flight had proven effective in reducing flight errors and accidents.

He ran into plenty of resistance, persevered, and eventually succeeded in creating simple steps that could be applied in any OR. Following these steps reduced the number of infections significantly, often to zero. In the process he changed elements of the way ORs function, moving from a Surgeon-is-God model to an OR-team-working-for-one-patient model. These efforts, reported in *Safe Patients, Smart Hospitals,* earned him a MacArthur Genius Award and opened the gates to more checklists and better group cohesion among medical teams.

Dr. Atul Gawande looks at many of these in *The Checklist Manifesto,* pointing out that something as simple as having an operating room team introduce themselves to one another before surgery begins can create a safer, more efficient environment.

Such lists may be DO-CONFIRM, where each member of a team handles certain elements and then confirms that they are complete when the group stops to go down the checklist together. Or they may be READ-DO, where one person reads the list aloud and everybody goes through each element of it together.

In both cases, they improve efficiency, and help explain why so many people want to take a look at your wrist ID band when you are hospitalized or undergoing an outpatient procedure. That's a step on all kinds of checklists, and a valuable one.

ARE ALL HOSPITALS THE SAME?

There are a number of different types of hospitals and where your sibling goes will depend on geography, the nature of her medical problem, provisions of her health insurance, and where her doctors are on staff.

The American Hospital Association compiles all manner of statistical information about hospitals, and their 2011 Annual Survey found 5,724 registered hospitals in the United States. These include all hospitals that meet AHA registration criteria, whether they belong to the AHA or not. Approximately 1,000 are investor-owned, for-profit institutions, another 1,200 are run by government entities, and about 3,000 are non-government, not-for-profit community hospitals.

So in theory at least, at least, over two-thirds of American hospitals are nonprofit. Remember that when you are trying to decipher a hospital bill with a bottom line the size of the GNP of a developing nation.

General or Community Hospitals are facilities of all sizes from teeny-weeny to gargantuan where medical and surgical patients are treated for a wide range of ailments. Usually there is an emergency room and sometimes a built-in ambulance service. General hospitals typically also have Intensive Care Units (ICUs) and laboratories.

Size isn't necessarily a determinant of excellence. A community hospital in St. Louis may be significantly larger than one a hundred miles away in a small Missouri town, but each is likely to handle the same sorts of cases, often with equal proficiency.

Teaching Hospitals are generally affiliated with a medical school, university, and/or nursing school. Frequently physicians on staff at teaching hospitals have highly specialized areas of practice and may be involved with research at the institution. Care is provided by a combination of licensed health care practitioners and students working under their supervision. The trade-off for having access to highly qualified physicians and diagnosticians at a teaching hospital may, however, be that you see a lot less of them and a lot more of the students.

Specialized Hospitals concentrate on one particular type of physical issue, such as children's or geriatric care, psychiatric care, rehabilitation, or a particular type of disease. Trauma centers also fall under this heading.

Clinics and Surgery Centers are more oriented toward outpatient treatment and are likely to be owned and operated by a private medical partnership or a governmental agency. Surgery Centers have expanded dramatically in the past few decades, sometimes so that the profits generated for specialty practices with a lot of outpatient procedures (e.g. colonoscopies) won't be diluted by sharing.

WHO PROVIDES THE CARE IN A HOSPITAL?

It is next to impossible to figure out who is who by their appearance in today's hospital, since traditional gender divisions no longer apply and many clinicians, technicians, and nurses wear similar uniforms. Almost none of those uniforms are white, either, though physicians may still wear the traditional white jacket.

You'll need to learn to read ID badges to keep track of the personnel.

Nursing staff consists of **Registered Nurses (RNs)**, **Licensed Practical Nurses (LPNs)**, and **Certified Nurse's Aides (CNAs)**. LPNs are known as **Licensed Vocational Nurses (LVNs)** in Texas and California, perhaps the only governmental policy the two states have in common. LPN/LVNs perform many of the same medical tasks as RNs, but don't make medical decisions. CNAs are associated more with personal care and non-medical routines. They work under the supervision of the others.

RNs have more extensive education than LVN/LPNs, but all must pass a national licensing exam. They are licensed by the states where they practice. LPNs sometimes get additional training to become RNs, and RNs in turn may go on to advanced degree programs and/or become nurse practitioners.

Medical Technicians may work entirely behind the scenes, but some interact directly with patients, often in conjunction with testing. Med techs run a lot of the diagnostic and treatment equipment in a hospital (e.g. X-rays and lab work) and often specialize. **Emergency Medical Technicians** (EMTs or paramedics) are a med tech variant, specializing in emergency stabilization and transport.

Larger hospitals or rehab facilities often have a **Social Worker** or **Case Manager** on site. These people can be extremely helpful in dealing with outside agencies if problems or complications occur, may be aware of local options you hadn't known about, and will also know how you can follow up once your sibling is discharged.

And don't forget the **Chaplain.** Any large facility will have at least one chaplain on the premises or nearby and if your sibling indicated a religious preference during admission, you're almost guaranteed a visit from somebody. This person may not be of precisely the same faith community as your sibling, but if what you want is somebody to pray over her or to pray with you, or to sit with you in the chapel for some respite, that service is generally available.

HOW CAN YOU PROTECT SOMEONE IN THE HOSPITAL?

The short answer here is "due diligence" and the unfortunate reality is that it is up to you to do everything possible to insure that your sibling is properly cared for.

This may involve what *doesn't* happen to her as much as what does. Since only seriously ill patients are kept overnight in hospitals these days, she is likely to be in no condition to pay attention to anything that needs to be watched.

If your sibling is going to be spending any length of time in a hospital or has a condition which may lead to a lengthy stay, I urge you to get hold of one of the patient checklist volumes listed at the end of this chapter. Hospitals are complicated places and these books will help you keep up with matters, though it's rarely possible to stay on top of everything in a fast-breaking medical adventure.

I am particularly fond of *Critical Conditions* by Martine Ehrenclou and *Hospital Stay Handbook* by Jari Holland Buck.

Both of these books grew out of the writers' personal experiences as loved ones went through an array of hospital experiences, and each shares a wealth of detailed and practical information gleaned from those experiences. *Critical Conditions* excels at very specific advice and offers plenty of checklists, with an emphasis on record-keeping. A significant portion of *Critical Conditions* consists of fill-in-the-blank sections designed to help you keep track of everything that is happening in a single, easily-accessed location.

Hospital Stay Handbook is set against the backdrop of the kind of medical horror story (complete with four different hospitals) that I normally wouldn't recommend to anybody who's ill, and it's even scarier since the hapless patient at its center was a doctor himself. But everything did eventually work out and he recovered, in no small measure due to the attention his advocate wife paid to every single detail.

The checklists are also excellent, and there's a little bonus woven through the book: a crash course in advocacy which will benefit anybody trying to take care of any medical problem, serious or otherwise.

HOSPITAL-ACQUIRED INFECTIONS

It's chilling to realize that hospital-acquired infections

are so common that they have their own acronym, HAI.

It's even more chilling to realize that the Centers for Disease Control estimate that 1.7 million people a year pick up HAIs and that somewhere between 50,000 and 100,000 of them die from them. Those figures are flexible (and probably low) because anybody in the hospital is already pretty sick and while an HAI may not be the outright cause of death, it can certainly push other afflictions over the edge.

These bugs purely love hanging out in hospitals where there are such easy pickings: weak, sick organisms, often with open pathways directly to the interior goodies. And there are ever so many places to hang out in hospitals! An opportunistic bug that hitches a ride on a blood pressure cuff or a food delivery cart, for instance, has the opportunity to visit all sorts of people in the course of a normal day.

There are a number of subcategories of these killer bugs, but the Big Three to be on guard against are MRSA (methicillin-resistant Staphylococcus aureus), pneumonia, and Clostridium difficile.

MRSA infections typically start on the skin. They spread fast and are resistant to many antibiotics, but are usually treatable so long as they are caught quickly. They can also lead to system-wide sepsis (blood poisoning) and death if not treated promptly and correctly.

Pneumonia may be the most commonly-acquired hospital-related infection, particularly among patients in ICU or on ventilators.

Clostridium difficile, or C diff, is an intestinal infection that often occurs when somebody has been on a lot of antibiotics. C diff ravages the digestive tract and is (as its name suggests) extremely difficult to treat.

If you notice serious or rapid changes in your hospitalized sibling's physical situation, tell somebody. Right away. Things to watch out for are fever, rapid heartbeat and breathing, rashes, and confusion.

Time matters.

WHAT ARE HOSPITALS DOING
ABOUT THESE INFECTIONS?

You would think that hospitals would be twisting their corporate selves into pretzels to stop making their patients sicker, and in a few cases you would be right. When hospitals become aggressively involved in combatting these problems, they are often extremely successful.

Perhaps the single most significant area that many hospitals are now addressing is hand washing. Yep, we're back to the childhood instruction to "wash your hands" and for the same reason: germs.

Hand-washing would seem to be a no-brainer, since people who work with sick people are in constant contact with germs in all kinds of unsavory ways. But perpetual handwashing is also hard on the hands, and staffs are often highly resistant to being told to do it. (Is anybody surprised that doctors are the most resistant of all?)

Extensive signage and instructions to wash for fifteen seconds—or through an entire round of "Happy Birthday"—aren't always effective, so some hospitals are now experimenting with RFID systems that offer gentle reminders akin to the beep of a cell phone if a doctor passes a sink and doesn't wash up. Hospitals have also discovered, to nobody's real surprise, that if you toss a bit of Big Brother into the mix via closed-circuit cameras or other electronic monitors, workers are much more likely to comply with hand-washing regulations.

Many hospitals and medical offices now have hand sanitizer dispensers displayed at regular intervals. Some also are using incentive programs (Wash your hands and get a pizza coupon!) and coworker coaches who enforce washing by issuing red cards to workers observed not washing correctly.

A recent study by the nation's largest hospital chain showed that following a specific decontamination regimen with 26,000 intensive care patients reduced the rate of bloodstream infections significantly. Since folks in ICU tend to be older and sicker and weaker than other patients, they are often the most vulnerable. These patients were given twice-daily antibacterial nose swabs and bathed daily with antiseptic wipes. And they didn't get as many bloodstream infections.

With a little luck, we'll be seeing this pattern repeated across the land. It also doesn't hurt that Medicare is starting to crack down on payment for preventable infections acquired in the hospital.

HOLIDAYS ARE NOT YOUR FRIEND

You will need to be exceptionally vigilant if your sibling's medical emergency occurs on or immediately before a holiday weekend. Medical personnel are on vacation or leaving, so they won't be around to follow up until Tuesday. Schedules are all switched around to accommodate coworkers and certain departments may be on skeleton staffs. ER staffs deal with unusually high numbers of amateur sports injuries and home-improvement mishaps, so they're particularly busy, even more so as the day wears on.

If you're scheduling surgery or a treatment, check the calendar and allow plenty of time before major holidays. You don't want to be worrying about complications setting in just as your doctor takes off for Fiji.

In his final four years, my brother had major medical incidents (strokes and grand mal seizures) on New Year's Day, Martin Luther King weekend (three times), Memorial Day weekend, Election Day, and shortly before both Easter and Christmas. I'm not sure how he happened to miss Labor Day, Thanksgiving, and the Fourth of July.

Everything took a little longer on those holiday weekends, and for most of them we didn't even have somebody on the spot, advocating for a dude who was not a very charming hospital patient and didn't believe there was anything really wrong with him. Even so, true emergency treatment was always provided well, we learned the ins and outs of distance emergency care, and we all got through it.

Just be prepared to wait longer for both care and information. And if you ever have the choice, get to the ER early in the day.

FIVE WAYS TO KEEP YOUR SIBLING SAFE IN THE HOSPITAL

1. Pay attention.

To everything. Make it your business to know what medications your brother is on and to notice when and how they're changed. Keep track of the equipment around the hospital bed and notice when something is changed. If things are supposed to be plugged in, make sure they are, particularly after cleaning people come in and out of the room.

Learn about scheduled treatments and tests, and mark surgical sites with a magic marker so nobody will get any surprises.

2. Get to know the people involved in your brother's care.

Come in to meet the primary doctor, specialist and/or hospitalist during rounds as soon as you can after your brother is admitted. It's worth going to some trouble to establish this connection and to determine what the best way and time will be for you to reach that doctor later to follow up. Doctors are notoriously hard to get hold of, as in "actually speak to." Have any questions or concerns written down so you won't forget.

Learn which nurses are involved in your brother's care and introduce yourself. Learn their schedules and shifts. Cultivate them all.

Communicate any particular concerns directly to these people. If your brother has a history of falls, make sure they know. If he's going to insist on trying to get into the bathroom on his own, tell them to watch out for that.

Be nice to all of these people. Very nice. Do your best to learn (and remember) their names and to smile when you see them, even if you're frantically distressed by your brother's condition. You don't have to like everybody, but it makes things easier—especially for the patient—if you at least pretend to.

This does not mean that you shouldn't speak up when something is amiss, or report somebody whose care you find unacceptable. That's why you're paying attention.

Use every possible opportunity to humanize your brother, particularly if he's not conscious or not himself. Talk about the work he does or used to do, his hobbies, his life—and bring in pictures for the bedside table, showing him at more vibrant moments. You want him to become Bob the Scoutmaster in their minds, not the cranky old goat in Room 413-2.

Critical Conditions suggests bringing in a box of candy or a tray of goodies for the nurse's station, with a note thanking them for taking such good care of your sibling. And be sure to firmly attach that note to the box or basket or tray, so everybody will know who's responsible.

3. Become a cleanliness fanatic.

Buy a pony keg of Purell and set it up on your brother's bedside table. Use it frequently yourself and ask anyone coming into the room to also use it. Ask with a smile, of course.

Bring in a container of antibacterial wipes and use them all around the room. Start with the bathroom and wipe any place anybody is likely to *ever* have touched. Get the bed rails and the bedside table and the tray table and the call button. Don't forget light switches and doorknobs and the arms on visitor chairs.

Do this regularly and thoroughly.

4. Keep your personal stuff out of the room.

Anything that you normally carry around and set down places—purse, backpack, briefcase—can serve as a transportation system for more bacteria to get into that room you've just been wiping down. Don't bring in food, don't eat in the sickroom, and don't put anything on the tray table. Leave the grandkids at home and don't even think about using the patient's bathroom.

5. Write it all down.

Have a notebook or a tablet or some other convenient way to keep track of what's going on and to easily retrieve information as needed. That info can be as simple as the names of the night shift nurses or as complicated as the historical changes in your brother's medications and medication schedule.

WHAT DO HOSPITAL
RANKINGS MEAN?

So you noticed there's a big banner hanging out in front of your local hospital, announcing that it is *The Best*.

Turns out that a whole lot of hospitals are the Best at something, but it isn't necessarily going to help you or your sibling one little bit. If a place is the best regional childbirth center and your brother has COPD, you'll want to go beyond the banner to find out if he really ought to be there in the first place.

Who designated the hospital as Best? Best at what? Look it up on the hospital's website, or ask at the Information Desk if your brother is already a patient. It ought to be easy to find this info, since hospitals tend to make a big deal out of it.

But keep in mind that inclusion on the "best" list—any best list—doesn't mean that this is the best place for him to be or that a specialty hospital is necessarily better at dealing with his condition than your local community hospital.

THE TOP HOSPITALS IN THE UNITED STATES

Having said all that, there are some very significant ratings that can be helpful, particularly if you are dealing with an unusual diagnosis and need to seek out more specialized care, either locally or farther afield if you live in the boonies.

For the 2015-16 ranking of the Honor Roll of Best Hospitals in the United States, *US News & World Report* looked at nearly 5,000 medical centers around the country and considered 16 medical specialties. If a hospital was designated as one of the best in six specialties or more, it made the Honor Roll. www./health.usnews.com/best-hospitals

HealthGrades is an independent rating system and it also has an Honor Roll, with entirely different criteria. No surprise, then, that the two lists are significantly different. HealthGrades looks at a wide range of different topics, including mortality rates, and is so comprehensive that its lists have lists. These can be accessed at www.healthgrades.com/quality/hospital-ratings-awards.

In addition to the Honor Roll list below, *US News & World Report* also ranks top hospitals in all of the specialties considered in creating the general list. Their lists are also broken down by metropolitan area. The criteria are fairly constant, and while hospitals may move up or down in a category, once they're on the list, they tend to stay on the list. Beyond the Honor Roll, specialty and metro area rankings can also be accessed.

US News & World Report's
2015-16 Hospital Honor Roll

1. Massachusetts General Hospital, Boston
2. Mayo Clinic, Rochester, New York
3. (tie) Johns Hopkins Hospital, Baltimore
3. (tie) UCLA Medical Center, Los Angeles
5. Cleveland Clinic, Cleveland
6. Brigham and Women's Hospital, Boston
7. New York-Presbyterian University Hospital of Columbia and Cornell, New York
8. UCSF Medical Center, San Francisco
9. Hospitals of the University of Pennsylvania-Penn Presbyterian, Philadelphia
10. Barnes-Jewish Hospital/Washington University, St. Louis
11. Northwestern Memorial Hospital, Chicago
12. NYU Longone Medical Center, New York
13. UPMC-University of Pittsburgh Medical Center
14. Duke University Hospital, Durham, North Carolina
15. Stanford Health Care-Stanford Hospital, California

HOSPITAL COSTS

This is the land of the $45 aspirin and it's far too complicated to get into here. The section on "Paying for It All" discusses this touchy issue, including information on how various elements of the health care community set their rates.

Hint #1: It's not to make things more affordable for the patient, even though a majority of hospitals in the United States are technically nonprofit.

Hint #2: Advertising the fact that a hospital is Best at Something costs big bucks, and they have to be passed on to somebody.

THE READMISSION BLUES

When you go home from the hospital, it's entirely reasonable to assume that you won't be back any time soon. Unfortunately that isn't always the case. People can and do get readmitted. Sometimes readmission is because a person is really ill and takes a turn for the worse, but sometimes they've just sent you home too soon. When you're readmitted, it costs everybody time and money—plus you're back in the hospital, where you didn't want to be in the first place.

Medicare is now penalizing hospitals with high readmission rates under a provision of the Affordable Care Act, the Hospital Readmission Reduction Program (HRRP). These penalties are financial.

On a more immediate and practical level, the best way to minimize the likelihood of readmission is to have somebody there and taking notes when your sibling is discharged. Listen carefully and ask questions. Don't assume that everything is covered in the wad of paper they will be handing you.

Make sure that you understand all instructions for care and don't leave without them. What doctor is your sibling supposed to follow up with and when? Have medications been changed and do new prescriptions need to be filled? Are there dietary changes, concerns, or restrictions? What should your sibling expect over the next few days?

Take your time. Ask as many questions as you need so that you understand what to do, what not to do, and what to watch out for.

BUT I'M NOT BETTER YET!

If your sibling is on Medicare and you believe that he is being discharged prematurely from the hospital or another care facility, you are entitled to something called "immediate advocacy" through Medicare Quality Improvement Organizations (QIOs). Call 1-800-MEDICARE or go to www.medicare.gov/ and search for QIO.

These reviews are handled by various agencies depending on the state you live in, and while they can't force a hospital to keep you, they can and do immediately get involved to try to find a mutually acceptable solution.

This system only works if a review of medical records is not required, and it's not a GET OUT OF PAYING card if you refuse to leave. But it will get an institution's attention, and often that's all that is necessary.

SHOULD YOU GO TO A
FANCY TEACHING FACILITY?

There comes a time in many serious illnesses when people start to think, "Maybe we ought to go to the Mayo Clinic." Or Sloan-Kettering or Johns Hopkins or Duke. And there are some instances where that is exactly the right thing to do—if you have the money and the time and the emotional wherewithal for everything that entails.

But going to a topnotch teaching facility isn't going to cure something that is incurable and there's often an aura of genuine desperation involved. You want a different answer. You want somebody to change the equation. You want your sister to live another twenty years.

Going to a high-end medical facility may make all the difference in the world. If you have a rare condition that's treated once a year at your local hospital and forty times a week at the fancy hospital, it's worth at least doing some research to see if going there is economically and technically feasible. One major obstacle may be the specifics of the patient's health insurance coverage. Another may be geography and the difficulty of travel when somebody is ill.

Just remember that this kind of medical help isn't necessarily going to be better. I'm thinking here of my doctor friend who spent a month at the Mayo clinic and still couldn't get a diagnosis. Or the physician husband of the author of *Hospital Stay Handbook,* whose worst experience was at a prestigious teaching hospital.

REHAB FACILITIES

"Rehab" is a word with radically different meanings even within the same general context, the medical world.

There's the rehab where people go to recover from various addictive behaviors that have gotten them in some kind of trouble, and it's the one we hear the most about, particularly when a wayward starlet or horny politician needs to shape up in a hurry.

Then there's the rehab where they send you when you aren't sick enough to stay in the hospital but you aren't well enough to go home yet, either. Where you go and how long you can stay in this sort of rehab are often a function of your health insurance.

These places really work at rehabilitation and at getting you in shape through physical, occupational, and speech therapy on a patient-by-patient basis. Patients often continue as outpatients after discharge.

While certain rehab facilities are specialized and limited to a particular type of medical problem, most have a mix of patients. Some patients may be there to become more comfortable with their new bionic knees while others are relearning basic skills to regain ground lost after a brain injury or stroke. There are often a few younger patients, generally recovering from auto and motorcycle crackups.

PET VISITS

This is, of course, absurdly obvious. People who have close relationships with their pets miss them a lot while they are hospitalized. This is particularly true of those who live alone, where both the two- and four-footed members of the partnership are codependents.

It can't exactly be characterized as a groundswell, but there are starting to be facilities scattered around the country which permit visits to long-term patients from their dogs. Everything is regulated like crazy, of course, but it works.

So far as I know, cats have not yet participated in this beta testing.

A TALE OF ONE HOSPITAL

In the late 1950s, the hospital where my father practiced on Chicago's South Side began to plan a new hospital out in the suburbs. In the corn fields, actually.

The Evangelical Hospital medical staff was hit up for donations and I'm pretty sure they all contributed through peer pressure, since much fuss was made about plaques honoring donors. Ground was broken in 1958 on farmland in Oak Lawn.

Christ Community Hospital opened in 1960 with 195 beds on four floors in a six-floor building. The top floors were finished and opened a couple years later; this was a cautious expansion into untested territory. For the first year, prior to accreditation, the hospital couldn't have its own interns, and staff doctors rotated being on call for the emergency room.

My father rented a two-room office in the basement and his contribution to the building fund was commemorated with a donor plaque on the door to the Doctors' Locker Room.

Some of my high school classmates were among the first students at the nursing school. An addition went up: three more floors in 1968. In 1970 when I was graduating from college, my father became Chief of Staff.

More buildings, more facilities, more parking. The bed

count kept rising and the services extending. It became a Level 1 Trauma Center and started work on a new emergency center and helipad to accommodate patients arriving from Chicago's violent and troubled South Side. My father moved his offices out of the basement to cushier and newer quarters upstairs and retired in the late 1980s.

Staff and consulting staff kept growing and new services and facilities kept opening: The Heart Institute for Children, a new emergency center, a Physicians Pavilion, a Surgery Pavilion, Hope Children's Hospital.

The name kept changing, too. First it was shortened to Christ Hospital. Then it was Christ Hospital and Medical Center, followed by EHS Christ Hospital and Medical Center. Its most recent name change and identity redesign came when it became Advocate Christ Medical Center in 2001, part of the Advocate Health Care system which operates a dozen hospitals in the Chicago area.

A couple years after that, a kid I've known since we went to church camp together in grade school became the Chief of Staff. My dad's old title.

Today Advocate Christ Medical Center has 694 beds and is one of the largest health care facilities in the Chicago area. The last time I drove by, construction was in full swing on a nine-story Outpatient Pavilion that looks like a Miami Beach hotel.

That website proudly proclaims all manner of (pardon the expression) cutting-edge technological services, including some I've never heard of. In 2011, the hospital had over 40,000 admissions and the emergency room saw nearly 250 patients every single day.

That's the same emergency service that one staff doctor could cover on call from his bedroom at home when the place first opened.

Oh, and it has all kinds of distinguished ratings from all kinds of organizations. These applaud excellence in treating an impressive range of medical problems and conditions. So I'm sure you won't be surprised to learn that Advocate Christ Medical Center is ranked by US *News & World Report* in the

Top Fifty nationwide for three adult specialties and one pediatric specialty.

All this and the place is barely fifty years old.

ADDITIONAL INFORMATION

American Hospital Association
www.aha.org

Healthgrades: Find a Doctor/Doctor Reviews/Hospital Ratings
www.healthgrades.com/

RID: Committee to Reduce Infection Deaths
www.hospitalinfection.org/

• • • • •

Elizabeth Bailey
The Patient's Checklist: 10 Simple Hospital Checklists to Keep You Safe, Sane & Organized
Sterling, 2012

Karen Curtiss
Safe & Sound in the Hospital: Must-Have Checklists and Tools for Your Loved One's Care
Partnerhealth, 2012

Jari Holland Buck
Hospital Stay Handbook: A Guide to Becoming a Patient Advocate for Your Loved Ones
Llewellyn Publications, 2007

Martine Ehrenclou
Critical Conditions: The Essential Hospital Guide to Get Your Loved One Out Alive
Lennon Grove Press, 2008

Atul Gawande
The Checklist Manifesto: How to Get Things Right
Picador, 2010

Marty Makary
Unaccountable: What Hospitals Won't Tell You and How Transparency Can Revolutionize Health Care
Bloomsbury, 2012

Maryanne McGuckin, Toni Goldfarb, Peter Pronovost
The Patient Survival Guide: 8 Simple Solutions to Prevent Hospital- and Healthcare-Associated Infections
Demos Health, 2012

Peter Pronovost and Eric Vohr
Safe Patients, Smart Hospitals: How One Doctor's Checklist Can Help Us Change Health Care from the Inside Out
Plume, 2011

Julie Salamon
Hospital: Man, Woman, Birth, Death, Infinity, Plus Red Tape, Bad Behavior, Money, God and Diversity on Steroids
Penguin, 2008

TREATMENT OPTIONS

There was a time, not all that long ago, when the doctor would brew you a nasty-tasting beverage from his herb garden and apply a few leaches.

Life is a little more complicated now.

It's likely that at some point—often early on—you will find yourself sorting through treatment options with the patient. Often these range from Unpleasant to God-awful, with intermediate stops at Painful, Humiliating, and Totally Debilitating.

If you're dealing with heart attack, stroke, recovery from an accident, or many types of surgery, the follow-up is likely to include all sorts of rehab: physical, occupational, psychological, speech. Dietary and exercise changes are usually recommended following a major cardiac event as well, and neither is generally greeted with much enthusiasm by the patient. Somebody whose idea of breakfast is eggs, bacon, sausage, home fries, and toast isn't going to greet a bowl of oatmeal or Greek yogurt with jubilation.

For cancer treatment, you will probably be looking at a combination of oncology and surgery, a package that often includes high doses of radiation and various cocktails of chemotherapy poisons. Completely apart from the question of whether these will actually work is the reality that for a while at least, the cure will be worse than the disease, which may have offered few outward symptoms at all before its discovery.

You may have never considered this illness or these treatment issues in terms of a sibling. Or maybe you have. Since so many diseases have genetic components, it's entirely possible that you've already been down some of the tributaries of this particular river with a parent, another sibling, or yourself.

If that's the case, you may already know way more than you ever wanted to about the familial affliction.

Not exactly a matter for congratulations, but it may save you enough time to slip in a good book or movie.

TYPES OF IMAGING

Advances in technology make it possible to locate and map tumors and other physical problems that once could only be guessed about without a surgical inspection. All of these methods fall in what used to be science fiction territory, using various types of rays and emissions and waves that cannot be seen as they work. They are far from interchangeable, and more recently developed techniques can be dramatically more expensive.

These types of imaging are used for diagnostic and tracking purposes. Don't confuse them with radiation therapy, commonly used as part of cancer treatment programs.

X-rays, the oldest member of this diagnostic family, have electromagnetic radiation for over a century to provide interior photographs of the body. These are typically two-dimensional, black-and-white negative pictures and are at their best when there is a sharp contrast between soft and hard tissues showing, for instance, a broken ankle or a decayed tooth.

Ultrasound (diagnostic sonography) is used to create images of soft tissues by mapping sound waves as they pass through the body. Sonograms create the fetal pictures that prospective parents pass around the office or post on social media. Ultrasound can also be used to determine what happens during certain soft-tissue processes, such as whether a bladder is emptying completely.

CT Scans (computerized tomography) create a series of cross sections of a part of the body to examine an organ or area in greater detail. Known as slices, these images create a three-dimensional picture of what may be amiss, or improving, or not there at all. About half of CT scans use radio contrast agents, and the machines whir while they're working, rotating around the patient's body.

MRI Scans (magnetic resonance imaging) provide better contrast resolution than CT scans, without using ionizing radiation. As its name suggests, this process uses magnetic force to create images in a sequence. MRI testing is noisy in a clattering kind of way and previously required being in a tightly enclosed area, a problem for claustrophobics. Open MRI equipment has now been developed, but if it's not available where you are, earplugs and light sedation may be in order.

PET Scans (positron emission tomography) create a multi-colored, 3-D view of the body and what is happening inside it. Primarily used to locate areas of metastasis or to track down a primary tumor in hiding, PET scanning provides a color image of the body's interior. The patient fasts prior to imaging so body cells are hungry, then is injected with radioactive glucose that is scarfed up by fast-growing cells that gobble the glucose and create bursts of light in the process. (Note: The physics is more complicated than this, as is often the case with physics.) 90% of PET scans are used to locate cancer metastasis.

SURGERY

While there have always been various types of treatments for illness—potions, medications, prayer—the rise of modern surgery has moved surgeons front and center, exactly where they like to be.

The development of modern anesthesia made it possible for doctors to open up the human body to see what problems existed and to correct them, often by removal of an organ or tumor. Today corrective surgery for all manner of physical problems sometimes begins *in utero* and may continue into a patient's tenth decade.

While surgery itself became more possible through anesthesia, survival of the surgical patient remained problematic.

Basic sanitation entered the operating room (and the hospital, for that matter) well after surgery became commonplace. Hand washing was optional and if a knife fell to the floor, the surgeon might just wipe it off and keep going. The development of proper antiseptic procedures represented a huge leap forward—Sterilization! Who'da thunk it?—and once antibiotics were discovered, all bets were off.

Anything that could be opened up, cleared out, exchanged for a better-functioning part, or otherwise corrected—surgery was on the job. The installation of factory-made hearts probably represented the peak of this surgical crescendo, though innovation certainly continues. New body parts are currently being created on 3-D printers, by special order.

Today's trend is toward less invasive surgery, often performed somewhere other than a hospital's operating room. Where a surgical patient might have languished for a week or two in the hospital when we were kids, you are now far more likely to be transferred from Recovery to your own car. Indeed, the rise of surgery centers completely removed from hospitals makes going home the only post-op option.

Operations which once required an abdominal incision are now often conducted using laparoscopy. This procedure—also called keyhole, Band-Aid, or minimally invasive surgery (MIS)—uses one or more very small incisions and then blows up the abdominal area with carbon dioxide like a flesh balloon. At that point, light and micro-instruments are inserted. By way of camera, the surgeon can see the organs displayed kind of like the Visible Man model with his transparent plastic skin. While this surgery is easier on the patient's body, the surgeon is unable to palpate organs and make decisions based on what they feel like, an important component of traditional surgery.

Robotic surgery is becoming more common for operations where access is difficult and precision is critical. Two types of surgery where this is common are brain and prostate. A surgeon controls and guides the robotic equipment. That surgeon is likely to be somebody who grew up on computers and long ago mastered gaming techniques.

Surgery is still used for cancer diagnosis in some cases, since technically the only certainty about something gone awry in the human body is what can be determined by examining its tissue with a biopsy. It may identify a type of tumor or determine the stage of a cancer. Occasionally cancer surgery is curative, and no further treatment is required, but that doesn't happen often. Sometimes oncologists prefer to shrink a tumor with radiation or chemotherapy before surgery, to make its size or location more manageable.

Location can be a problem if something is cozied up to a very important organ or nerve or whatever. When a tumor is declared to be inoperable, it's generally because of its location and the potential for greater harm in trying to remove it. In this case, the tumor may be debulked, removing as much of it as possible.

Certain specialized surgical techniques are used in particular treatments, often named for the originating surgeon. One example is the Whipple procedure for pancreatic cancer, and another is Mohs surgery for skin cancers.

THE HISTORY OF
BREAST CANCER TREATMENT

Perhaps nothing illustrates the changing role of surgery in modern medicine better than the treatment of breast cancer.

Early surgical treatment for cancer aimed at getting as much of the tumor as possible, while checking to see visually if it had already spread. It was believed then that this spreading moved like sound waves, radiating outward from the tumor.

The radical mastectomy has been around in some form for millennia, but the modern version was developed around the turn of the 20th Century. This operation removed the tumor, the breast, and quite a lot of surrounding flesh, well up into the armpit and sometimes including ribs in its truly radical days. (Some of these operations were performed before anesthesia. Women are tough.)

The radical mastectomy was also a very immediate procedure, in the belief that not a minute could be wasted. As quickly as possible after a lump was discovered, surgery was scheduled. The patient going under anesthesia didn't know whether she'd wake up with one breast or two.

During surgery, a biopsy would be taken and sent to Pathology, where a frozen section of the tumor was examined under a microscope by a pathologist.

If the pathologist saw cancer cells, surgery would continue immediately.

As a teenager contemplating a medical career, I once spent a day in the Pathology Lab at my father's hospital and saw this process firsthand. The specimen was rushed down from Surgery, then flash-frozen, sliced, and observed. The diagnosis was cancer. Half an hour later, a steel pan containing the woman's breast came down to the lab.

Today's breast cancer surgical patient is less rushed and faces a wide range of less-invasive options, beginning with lumpectomy. (Which, as it happens, was suggested back in the late 1920s and pooh-poohed by the surgical establishment.) Reconstructive surgery is a given and may begin during the initial operation.

OTHER CANCER TREATMENTS

Treatment plans beyond (and including) surgery are a huge part of cancer management. These vary widely depending on the type of cancer and when it was diagnosed. Some types of cancer are a whole lot worse than others, and in general, the further a cancer has advanced, the tougher it is to treat or cure.

The thing to keep in mind here is that cancer treatment is really, really hard on the body. And your sibling's body was already doing its best to fight off the cancer when medical science got involved, so it wasn't at its prime even before the diagnosis.

Your brother's type of tumor may have very standard, time-tested protocols or there may be ongoing controversy over which of several options is best. Whatever the treatment, it is likely to include any or all of the three standard prongs: surgery, radiation, chemotherapy. The order of these may vary.

The American Cancer Society website has exhaustive information on every conceivable kind of cancer treatment, including complementary and alternative (nontraditional) methods. Any idea about the treatment of cancer that you might ever have heard of will probably turn up here, along with a whole lot of things that may have you shaking your head. Remember laetrile? www.cancer.org/treatment/

The cliché is that cancer treatments are often far worse than the symptoms of the disease itself, that you have to make people sicker to make them better, and that oncologists will keep trying things until you recover, die, or refuse further treatment.

Like so many clichés, this one is solidly grounded in truth.

RADIATION THERAPY

Radiation treatment is designed to burn away rapidly growing cancer cells, just like something out of a superhero comic book.

ZAP!

The problem is that rays powerful enough to annihilate cancer cells are also very hard on anything else they might happen to hit. You don't want to burn away important, useful tissue while you're zapping a tumor.

Here's where all that imaging comes in. It's used to identify the precise location of the area to be zapped, and to figure out the best angles to reach the tumor without hurting anything else. A robot is programmed with this information and moves around the patient, delivering precise and predetermined radiation. It hits exactly the same spots from exactly the same angles every day you are in treatment.

This precision is assured by the creation of special masks or molds to hold the body in exactly the right place. Tattoos may also be used to map out an area of assault.

Treatment protocols vary but generally consist of a lengthy period of daily treatment, with weekends off for recuperation. Recuperation is necessary because radiation therapy drains energy dramatically. Appetite diminishes or vanishes and food races through the digestive system. Pounds melt away, sometimes the same ones you've been fighting to get rid of for years.

And you're tired. Really, really tired, requiring naps and more hours of sleep at night than you recall ever needing before.

This may or may not get better over time.

I remember being puzzled by how tired my brother seemed to be, years after his treatment for a malignant brain tumor, and being unable to find any information on the topic. (This was in the mid-90s, before widespread Internet access.) Finally, in a series of tapes ordered from a brain tumor conference, I found the answer: radiation. Actually, it was an extrapolation more than an answer, since it turned out there wasn't a sufficiently large group of long-term brain tumor survivors to study.

So they looked instead at breast tumor survivors, far greater in number, and determined that a certain percentage remained fatigued indefinitely.

CHEMOTHERAPY

The thing to remember about chemotherapy is that it is the intentional poisoning of a human organism. Everything else that happens—the good, the bad, the ugly—stems from that essential truth.

Chemotherapy regimens are constantly being changed and improved, improvement being gauged by how effectively they work in annihilating or reducing the malignancy. Sometimes chemo can completely eradicate a tumor. Sometimes it can't. What works in one patient with a particular cancer may not work in another.

Nor is there any consistency in the types of treatments. Sometimes it's slow infusions lasting several hours in a reclining chair at a medical facility and sometimes it's a single, gazillion-dollar pill that you take at home. The American Cancer Society website lists hundreds of different treatments, along with extensive information on each. www.cancer.org

Some types of chemo are immediately debilitating and others sneak up on the patient, sometimes over the course of several rounds. A chemo protocol may go on for a year or more if that is what's currently believed to be the optimal treatment for a particular type of cancer.

CHEMO BRAIN

When people talk about "chemo brain," they refer to a general cognitive fuzziness that a number of chemotherapy patients have noticed. It even has a fancy name: post-chemotherapy cognitive impairment (PCCI). This is not uncommon among many people undergoing chemotherapy, but it can linger in others. These are more likely to be people under treatment for reproductive-related cancers.

IMMUNOTHERAPY

Immunotherapy is based on the notion that the best tool in fighting cancer may be your own body's immune system. The challenge is to access that system and get it to perform as desired.

White blood cells may be removed and reprogrammed, or something called PD blockers may be employed. The goal is to get past the built-in protections that cancer uses to keep your body's immune system from immediately getting on the job.

For the most part, immune therapy is still considered breaking news, though I recently read about a man whose brain tumor, a deadly Glioblastoma, has not returned for two years after being directly infused with polio virus after pre-op Salk vaccination. The body set to work wiping out the polio virus and took the brain tumor with it. He didn't contract polio either.

This would seem to explain something that happened early in my brother's brain tumor treatment. Shortly after his initial surgery, he developed an infection in his brain that required a second operation. At the time, medical personnel said that such infections sometimes prevent the tumor from returning.

And while he developed many other problems related to that tumor over the final eighteen years of his life, the tumor itself never did came back.

ORTHOPEDIC SURGERY

There are all kinds of creative and dramatic ways to break bones when you're a kid, and if you're nodding your head at this sentence, you probably had more than one cast signed by classmates.

If you *don't* have a history of broken bones, however, encountering the world of orthopedic surgery as an adult in advanced middle age can be a sobering experience. Older people break bones in falls or vehicular accidents. Repairing those breaks can be a lot more complicated than the session you remember from your childhood ER, where the doctor adjusted your arm, took an X-ray, and sent you home in five pounds of plaster.

There is some uncertainty about whether older people who wind up on the ground with a broken bone either (a) fell and broke that bone, or (b) fell because that bone weakened and broke. All pretty chicken-or-egg, actually, since either way the bone is broken.

Orthopedic surgery is often required for seniors to make sure that the bone ends (and pieces; elderly bones shatter more easily than young resilient ones) are exactly where they ought to be to maximize healing. Methods of immobilization are more lightweight these days, occasionally removable, and sometimes available in hot pink or purple.

These breaks take longer to heal than when you were a kid and may require physical therapy. They may also require inpatient rehab, particularly if stairs are part of the patient's living setup or if the patient lives alone. While healing, your sister may need to use some combination of crutches, walkers, braces, and canes. Maybe even a wheelchair. This is all extremely annoying, of course, but there are some innovations to make it easier, like a one-sided kneeling crutch that allows you to use both hands while standing.

JOINT REPLACEMENTS

Even if you don't fall, you may still require orthopedic surgery if your joints are starting to wear out. People who require joint replacements range from lifelong jocks to the perpetually sedentary.

The good news is that they're cranking out plenty of bionic joints, and those replacements—made of plastic, ceramic, or metal—are designed to improve upon the worn-out parts they replace. The bad news is that these joints can be very expensive.

And it goes without saying that you'll be needing physical therapy to get that joint working in synch with the rest of the body.

REHAB

This is not the kind of rehab where wayward starlets learn how to make their own beds for five grand a day while trying to kick a cocaine habit. Substance abuse is a different animal and will be discussed later.

This is old-fashioned rehabilitation and it comes in a wide range of sizes, shapes, and colors, depending on what the original medical problem might be and how other treatment has improved (or in some cases temporarily worsened) the patient's original condition. Its goal and purpose are the same in all cases: to help the patient resume an approximation of the life she was previously leading.

Physical therapy is common after many types of orthopedic surgery, including joint replacements. It may also be necessary to rebuild damaged neural pathways following a stroke or other brain incident. A motivated patient will probably be able to continue this type of rehab independently with a gym membership or on home exercise equipment, after you dig it out of a basement corner.

Speech therapy may be required after a stroke or other major brain event.

Occupational therapy works to get the patient back to where she was in terms of performing tasks that may once have been routine, such as small motor skills that may need to be regained.

All of these are enormously frustrating, since what the patient is trying to regain are matters that once were routine, like talking or walking or pouring a beer. Whether inpatient, outpatient, or independent, all types of rehab are enhanced by the efforts of a motivated patient who is working to improve. It's useful to have supportive family members and friends around for this, as a reminder that progress *is* being made, however slowly.

A patient undergoing intensive rehab needs all the Attaboys or Attagirls you can come up with. And a whole bunch more on top of that. Think in terms of small rewards for any kind of progress: a favorite meal, a favorite DVD, chocolate, or flowers of any sort.

ALTERNATIVE MEDICAL TREATMENTS

At some point or another in almost any serious medical situation, somebody is going to bring up alternative treatment options. That person might even be you.

Many people swear by holistic treatments, acupuncture, massage therapy, megavitamins, specialized equipment, and the tenets of tribal medical practices from around the globe. A lot of these things work, though traditional physicians tend to shake their heads and mutter, "Cluck, cluck" when you bring them up.

If the person who wants to pursue an alternative treatment is the patient and you are a firm believer in 21st Century Medicine, keep in mind that *you are not the patient*. If there is a tried-and-true medical treatment that your sister does not want to consider and you are positive it will save her life, by all means encourage her to make that decision. But if she is determined to follow a different path, it's her call and you should respect that decision.

It may work, after all, and if it doesn't, you'll be there to assist her back onto the path you prefer while administering a hearty dose of "I told you so." Just like when you were kids.

Don't automatically scoff at alternative medicine. It's the only option that people in many parts of the globe have, and it becomes less threatening with familiarity.

When President Nixon visited China for the first time in 1972, a member of the press corps underwent an emergency appendectomy, an event which passed into the public consciousness as one using acupuncture for both anesthesia and pain management. When I looked up that event just now, it turns out that the reporter's situation was more medically complicated than that, but acupuncture (and its needle-free cousin, acupressure) are now considered perfectly acceptable treatment options by many in the US.

Lots of people use and swear by supplements of all sorts, ranging from a chewable multivitamin to eye of newt. Keep in mind that **these are all medications**. If your sibling is taking supplements of any kind, her health care team needs to know about it. That includes vitamins and minerals as well as less traditional brews.

Many holistic treatments have the potential to counteract conventional medication, or to expand its effectiveness to life-threatening levels. Natural drugs are drugs, whether they're freshly-cut leaves for chewing or have been distilled into gel caps. Just because it costs a lot and comes from the health food store or your neighbor's private dispensary (or holistic formulary) doesn't necessarily make it safe.

Alternative medicine may perform miracles, but it does not always work out as well as people hope. Ask Steve Jobs.

EXTREMELY UNCONVENTIONAL
TREATMENTS

Sometimes things are not going well at all with traditional treatments and a patient is getting worse. This is the point at which people begin considering less orthodox treatment possibilities.

If things are really grim and your brother wants to take a shot at something you consider out-and-out lunacy, it's his body and his illness.

You may, however, point out to him that world history has been liberally sprinkled with medical charlatans. Government approval of medical regimens and treatments can sometimes take frustratingly (even fatally) long periods of time, but there is generally not a conspiracy to keep a legitimate drug from reaching patients who need it, a common claim of many contemporary snake oil salesmen.

(Note: Just because a claim is made in a full-page ad in a reputable publication doesn't make it legitimate. Advertising's goal is to sell product, not truth.)

Every successful conventional treatment was an innovation at some point, of course, and new ones are being developed all the time. But I urge you to exercise caution with a treatment when you aren't able to find a record of it anywhere except with the person selling it.

When something sounds too good to be true—well, we all know how that's likely to end.

TREATMENTS FOR DEMENTIA AND ALZHEIMER'S

Alzheimer's accounts for 60-80% of those diagnosed with dementia, and the vascular dementia that occurs in some post-stroke patients is the second most common among a number of other forms of similar dementias. The word dementia itself has some unfortunate associations—as in *demented*, or just plain crazy—but it's more accurate and inclusive.

Alzheimer's is progressive and degenerative, has become more and more prevalent, and shows no signs whatsoever of slowing down. Nor have we seen a lot of developments in early diagnosis, treatment, or medication, though a number of medications and treatments may slow down the disease or deal with particular behavioral situations that it creates.

So far, however, there's been nothing significant in the area of reversal, which is pretty damned depressing considering that over 5 million people have Alzheimer's right now, a number that's projected to hit 7.1 million by 2025.

Still, a lot of scientists are working overtime.

Recent studies suggest links to such possible causes and contributing factors as heavy metals (particularly that bad boy copper), diabetes, hypertension, uncontrolled high cholesterol, anemia, early retirement, head injuries, obesity, and depression. When you look at a list like that, of course, it seems pretty clear that everything but ingrown toenails is a risk factor.

Good news, however, for cancer patients and survivors: A study of 3.5 million veterans discovered that those diagnosed with most cancers were not as likely to develop Alzheimer's at any point in life, and that chemotherapy strengthened the dementia shield.

Treatment at the moment is limited and plenty of highly-touted new drugs have failed at the clinical trial level.

A class of drugs called cholinesterase inhibitors— donepezil (Aricept); galantamine (Razadyne); rivastigmine (Exelon); and tacrine (Cognex)—are often prescribed to temporarily slow symptoms, but at least half of the people treated don't show any improvement and tacrine has fallen out of favor because of liver damage side effects.

Memantine (Namenda) is an NMDA (N-methyl-D-aspartate) antagonist that functions differently and may be more effective if taken with a cholinesterase inhibitor. These drug combinations may buy time, but not nearly enough.

As the disease takes hold, medications may become necessary for behavioral problems and issues. These include antidepressants, anti-anxiety drugs, and antipsychotics.

Experimentation continues on many other fronts, including deep brain stimulation like that sometimes used in treatment of Parkinson's disease and other movement disorders. One bright (or at least brightish) spot is that the US Food and Drug Administration (FDA) intends to ease approval rules to bring new therapies to patients more quickly.

A potential pre-emptive approach to treatment comes through a recently-announced grant to investigate whether it is possible to delay cognitive problems in people known to have a genetic predisposition to Alzheimer's.

Alzheimer's seems like it ought to be a simple fix, and maybe it is. One day we may wake up to find that the mystery has been solved overnight and that a full Alzheimer's cure (or vaccination) requires only a single dose of some oddball herb easily propagated in any home garden.

And wouldn't that be sweet?

GETTING BETTER
CUSTOMER SERVICE

Many types of treatment involve repeat visits to one or more medical facilities. If you are taking a sibling for treatment and the facility is particularly grim, be proactive. Pick up a potted plant at the grocery store, take it in, and present it to the staff with thanks for the good service your sister is getting.

If the service hasn't actually been that great, you may shame them into paying better attention to her. And even if it's already terrific, the staff will be grateful that you noticed. If you can afford it, bring a new plant each week and maybe some of them will survive to cheer on future patients once your sister is all better. By all means re-gift well-intentioned food items, too. If somebody brought her cookies that she can't eat because of nausea, put them on a nice paper plate and bring them in for the staff room at the chemo center.

I once had a student who wrote a memorable essay about positive attitude during her chemotherapy. She thanked everybody she dealt with every time she went in for chemo and she always brought flowers. I thought at the time that she was clearly a better person than I am. I still think so, and I really admire her approach.

Nobody needs to turn into a suffocatingly cheerful Pollyanna, but an occasional smile and a little potted ivy can go a long way.

PALLIATIVE CARE

Palliative care is sometimes confused with hospice care, but the reality is that they are far from interchangeable.

Hospice care concerns end of life treatments.

Palliative care treats the symptoms of an illness at any point, without necessarily treating or even acknowledging the illness itself. For example, somebody with acute migraines may take painkillers which ease the symptoms without addressing causation or cure of the actual migraines.

Palliative care may also be used in conjunction with other therapies, to ease symptoms of either the disease or its treatments. A classic example is the use of marijuana to ease nausea in chemotherapy patients or to enhance appetite in AIDS patients. (Medical marijuana will be discussed in the chapter on "Medications.")

Palliative care doesn't need to be medicinal, either. It can be as simple and rewarding as a nice massage or a luxurious bubble bath.

CLINICAL TRIALS

At some point you may want to look into experimental protocols, also known as clinical trials. The good news is that there are plenty of ongoing treatment trials for all sorts of diseases. The bad news is that these are usually blind studies, where you might be getting the potential miracle drug but may just as easily receive the placebo: a very fancy sugar pill.

One major consideration is the nature of the illness. If it's something progressive like Parkinson's or MS, there's time to think through the consequences of participation. But if you're dealing with a fast and deadly form of cancer, one that hasn't been responding well to treatment, you may need to roll the dice in a hurry.

The likelihood of finding something local and convenient improves dramatically if you happen to live in an area where a lot of medical research goes on. Generally, this means metropolitan areas with science-strong universities and/or teaching hospitals, often grouped in informal uber-medical clusters. If you're really, really sick, it doesn't hurt to be in Boston.

It's also possible that there's a whole lot of nothing going on in your geographical area related to your sister's disease. In that case, you may be looking at relocation to the research area for a period of time, with all of the obvious complications that kind of situation creates.

There's an element of lottery in this as well.

Things could go very well. Somebody is going to be in the clinical trial that leads to the cure for any disease, and it just might be your sister. Also, the results of a trial are occasionally so striking that researchers cut it off midway so everybody can get the wonder drug, though this doesn't happen often. The flip side, also infrequent, is that a trial may also be abruptly stopped if unexpected adverse reactions occur.

Encourage your sister to think it through carefully.

Does she really want to do this? Is it worth going halfway across the country to participate in some study when she is likely to die anyway—and would rather do so at home? Ideally, you want to balance the potential unpleasantness of the projected treatment against the reasonable expectation of improved health or additional life.

Will she be submitting to six months of hell for something that will only buy her another six months? Or, even worse, won't buy her anything if she gets the sugar pill? Too many treatments for too many illnesses play this terrible medical zero-sum game.

Which leads to an unfortunate fact of life: Generally, patient admission to these kinds of clinical trials is granted only after every other reasonable treatment has failed. At this point, your sister is likely to be really, really sick. When you have no remaining treatment options, any odds of getting the potential miracle drug sound pretty good.

You should also keep in mind that people may not be accepted into clinical trials if they are still being treated with conventional therapy. This doesn't mean that you *can't* get into a trial, but it does cut back on the likelihood.

WHERE YOU CAN FIND
CLINICAL TRIALS

For cancer trials, the National Cancer Institute features current information on clinical trials, and recently listed 12,000 of them.
www.cancer.gov/about-cancer/treatment/clinical-trials/search
You can also find information on clinical trials for specific types of cancers on their individual websites and from the American Cancer Society.
www.cancer.org/treatment/treatmentsandsideeffects/clinicaltrials/index
Numerous dementia clinical trials around the country can be located on the Alzheimer's Foundation website at www.alzfdn.org/ClinicalTrials/findatrial.html
or the Alzheimer's Association website at www.alz.org/research/clinical_trials/find_clinical_trials_trialmatch.asp.
Parkinson's clinical trial information is available through the Michael J. Fox Foundation www.foxtrialfinder.michaeljfox.org/
Many other disease websites offer information on clinical trials related to those diseases. If you can't find information there, try calling the 800 number and asking where you can get specifics.
www.cancer.gov/about-cancer/treatment/clinical-trials/search

MEDICAL TOURISM

For years I was aware that people in Southern California with major dental problems often went to Mexico where they could get treatment at considerably less cost than at home.
Well, medical tourism isn't just for toothaches any more.

People are scurrying around the globe, having joints replaced, and new kidneys installed, and all sorts of procedures performed.

For the most part, this is economic. Insurance policies may not cover joint replacements, for instance, or may do so with gargantuan deductibles. In that case it can actually be cheaper and easier to get that hip replaced abroad.

Medical tourism is not for everybody. You need to be comfortable traveling, to start with, and willing to spend a period of time in a country you may never have visited before. Give yourself fifteen bonus points if you speak the language in that country. Do your homework. Figure out the consequences. Get travel insurance.

Medical tourism carries inherent risks, but you may just end up paying a fraction of what it would have cost to replace that hip or take care of some other problem, with splendid and healthy results.

ADDITIONAL INFORMATION

Cancer Treatment

American Association for Cancer Research
www.aacr.org
866.423.3965

American Cancer Society
www.cancer.org
800.227.2345

Association of Cancer Online Resources (Information Sharing Communities)
www.acor.org/

National Cancer Institute at the National Institutes of Health (Clinical Trials)
www.cancer.gov
800.4.CANCER

•••••

American Cancer Society
Complete Guide to Complementary and Alternative Cancer Therapies, 2nd Edition
American Cancer Society, 2009

American Cancer Society
Guide to Pain Control, Revised Edition
American Cancer Society, 2004

Jeanne Besser, Kristina Ritley, Sheri Knecht, Michele Szafranski
What To Eat During Cancer Treatment: 100 Great-Tasting, Family-Friendly Recipes to Help You Cope
American Cancer Society, 2009

Abby S. Bloch, Barbara Grant, Kathryn K. Hamilton, Cynthia A. Thomson, eds.
American Cancer Society Complete Guide to Nutrition for Cancer Survivors: Eating Well, Staying Well During and After Cancer, 2nd Edition
American Cancer Society, 2010

Linda Carlson and Michael Speca
Mindfulness-Based Cancer Recovery: A Step-by-Step MBSR Approach to Help You Cope with Treatment and Reclaim Your Life
New Harbinger Publications, 2011

Ellen Clegg and Stewart Fleishman
ChemoBrain: How Cancer Therapies Can Affect Your Mind
Prometheus, 2009

Joanne Frankel Kelvin and Leslie Tyson
100 Questions & Answers About Cancer Symptoms and Cancer Treatment Side Effects
Jones and Bartlett, 2011

National Cancer Institute, National Institutes of Health, US Department of Health and Human Services
Eating Hints: Before, During and After Cancer Treatment
CreateSpace, 2012

National Cancer Institute
Facing Forward: Life After Cancer Treatment
Amazon Digital Services, 2011

National Cancer Institute, National Institutes of Health, US Department of Health and Human Services
Chemotherapy and You: Support for People with Cancer
CreateSpace, 2012

Dan Silverman and Idelle Davidson
Your Brain After Chemo: A Practical Guide to Lifting the Fog and Getting Back Your Focus
Da Capo, 2009

Connie Strasheim
Defeat Cancer: 15 Doctors of Integrative and Naturopathic Medicine Tell You How
BioMed Publishing, 2011

US Department of Health and Human Services and National Institutes of Health
Chemotherapy and You: Support for People with Cancer
Porch ePublishing, 2012

US Department of Health and Human Services and National Institutes of Health
Radiation Therapy and You: Support for People with Cancer
Amazon Digital Services, 2012

Clinical Trials

Clifton Leaf
"Do Clinical Trials Work?" *The New York Times,* July 13, 2013

Surgery

Marina S. Kurian, Barbara Thompson, and Brian K. Davidson
Weight Loss Surgery for Dummies, 2nd Edition
Dummies Books, 2012

Steven L. Orebaugh
Understanding Anesthesia: What You Need to Know About Sedation and Pain Control
Johns Hopkins Press, 2011

Amy L. Sutton, ed.
Surgery Sourcebook, 3rd Edition
Omnigraphics Health Reference Series, 2013

Paul Whang
Operating Room Confidential: What Really Goes on When You Go Under
ECW Press, 2010

Treatment Issues

Alan Zelicoff
More Harm Than Good: What Your Doctor May Not Tell You About Common Treatments and Procedures
AMACOM, 2008

Treatment Alternatives

Stephen Harrod Buhner
Herbal Antibiotics: Natural Alternatives for Treating Drug-Resistant Bacteria, 2nd Edition
Storey Publishing, 2012

William Collinge
The American Holistic Health Association Complete Guide to Alternative Medicine
Grand Central Publishing, 2009

Larry Malerba
Green Medicine: Challenging the Assumptions of Conventional Health Care
North Atlantic Books, 2010

Mayo Clinic
Book of Alternative Medicine, 2nd Edition
Oxmoor House, 2010

Earl Mindell and Virginia Hopkins
Prescription Alternatives: Hundreds of Safe, Natural, Prescription-Free Remedies to Restore and Maintain Your Health, 4th Edition
McGraw-Hill, 2009

Paul A. Offit
Do You Believe in Magic? The Sense and Nonsense of Alternative Medicine
Harper, 2013

Amy L. Sutton, ed.
Complementary and Alternative Medicine Sourcebook, 4th Edition
Omnigraphics Health Reference Series, 2010

Larry Trivieri and John W. Anderson, eds.
Alternative Medicine: The Definitive Guide, 2nd Edition
Celestial Arts Press, 2013

Medical Tourism

Paul Gahlinger
The Medical Tourism Travel Guide: Your Complete Reference to Top-Quality, Low-Cost Dental, Cosmetic, Medical Care & Surgery Overseas
Sunrise River Press, 2008

Patrick W. Marsek and Frances Sharpe
The Complete Idiot's Guide to Medical Tourism
Idiot Guides, 2009

George Puckett
Mexico-Medical/Dental Tourism
ESP Media, 2012

Stephanie Watson and Kathy Stolley
Medical Tourism (Contemporary World Issues)
ABC-CLIO, 2012

Josef Woodman
Patients Beyond Borders: Everybody's Guide to Affordable, World-Class Medical Travel
Healthy Travel Media, 2009

MEDICATIONS

Ask your doctor if medical advice from a television commercial is right for you.

—Bumper sticker

We've all seen the ads.

Silver-haired couples walking hand-in-hand toward the bedroom after the gentleman has taken a pill that will have his lady in ecstasy for hours. Sixty-somethings rediscovering the joys of eating without gastric distress, sleeping like newborns, avoiding random leakage, exercising exuberantly without fear of springing a hamstring or loosening a sphincter.

We've all heard the voice-over warnings, too.

Lists of complications that could fell entire counties, dire warnings about the hundred horrible things that might happen if you take this pill, and always the obligatory caution that yes, this drug could kill you—though death is not really all that common.

This advertising does not appear as a public service.

Pharmaceutical companies (AKA Big Pharma) pay big bucks for ads to tout newly developed medications because they want you to pester your doctor to prescribe them and solve all your problems. And maybe your doctor will.

Maybe your doctor would have suggested these medications anyway. Big Pharma has also been working overtime behind the scenes.

And let's be fair. That medication may be just the breakthrough you've been waiting years for. Every incredible medical breakthrough has to start somewhere.

WHAT ARE DRUGS?

American pharmaceuticals are chemical compounds

created under laboratory conditions, tested first on animals and then on human beings. Big Pharma then brings them to the marketplace for sale through licensed pharmacies, when prescribed to specific patients by licensed physicians.

Which sounds simple enough, right? Drugs are whatever you need a prescription for.

Except that other things are drugs, too.

Vitamins and minerals in tablet or liquid form. Herbs in pills, compounds, compresses, salads, or tea. Endorphins produced by an enthusiastically-exercised brain. Tobacco, alcohol, and caffeine. Not to mention illicit and/or recreational drugs, many of which are also legitimate drugs under different circumstances.

So let's go with the Wikipedia definition here: *A drug is a substance which may have medicinal, intoxicating, performance enhancing or other effects when taken or put into a human body or the body of another animal and is not considered a food or exclusively a food.*

The drugs that are produced by Big Pharma are not sent out into the marketplace primarily to promote the common good and create better health, though everybody loves it when that happens. They are sent out to make money.

Whatever else happens are side effects.

PATENTED DRUGS

Like other inventions, new drugs can be patented. Developing new pharmaceuticals is an expensive and time-consuming process, one with far more failures than successes. In order to recoup all those research and development expenses, Big Pharma sometimes prices new drugs at levels that can be real budget busters. We'll get to that later.

A drug may be **patented** at any stage of development, with the patent lasting twenty years from the time of filing, though like most things associated with the pharmaceutical industry, this is often more complicated. The US Patent and Trademark Office handles patents for drugs, along with widgets, space shuttles, and that wacky little thing your neighbor devised for finding his lost golf balls.

A slightly different issue is **exclusivity,** which is handled by the Food and Drug Administration (FDA). Exclusivity generally lasts no longer than seven years and may be much shorter. It's designed to protect the interests of a drug manufacturer from immediate copycat production. This is covered in great detail at www.fda.gov/Drugs/ and is also exceedingly complicated.

And in case that wasn't confusing enough, some drugs have never been patented or exclusive at all.

GENERIC DRUGS

The biggest problem with generic drugs is their name.

"Generic" just sounds cheap, not to mention vaguely disreputable. You know, like those black-and-white cans labeled "Corn" that food manufacturers once tried to market as affordable alternatives to products with pretty pictures on the labels.

Lots of people (and nearly half of all physicians!) believe that generic drugs do not have reliable quality. There does not seem to be scientific evidence to back this up. Indeed, Big Pharma has a lot at stake in having fewer generics around, so you have to figure that if there were real problems, we'd be hearing about them.

The irony of generic drugs is that often the people who most benefit financially from using them consider it a form of discrimination, a way of foisting inferior medications on the poor. Meanwhile, on the other side of the tracks, savvy consumers of more comfortable means regard generics more accurately as a rare bargain in the medical world.

Generic drugs are identical reproductions of patented drugs, bioequivalent to the medications they replicate. Not all patented drugs become generic, however, if there isn't sufficient demand to justify the cost of producing and testing to bring out a generic.

But if something is popular or particularly good at what it does, other manufacturers will want to get into the act when its patent expires. First the FDA must approve their products, under an abbreviated process, to be sure that they *are* identical. (Note: Inert ingredients in the original drug do not have to be replicated and may differ, which is also true for generic over-the-counter drugs. Occasionally this creates problems for those with sensitivities to those inert ingredients.)

However, simply because a generic is available does not mean that it is actually *available*. Purchasing organizations which control the acquisition of drugs, supplies, and devices for health care facilities sometimes make sweetheart deals with vendors. If such a deal is made with a single generic vendor, for instance, you'd better hope that vendor has enough to meet that order and still take care of you.

Despite all the obstacles, however, 84 percent of prescriptions filled in the United States in 2012 were for generic drugs. Many insurance companies, the Veterans Administration, and a number of states require that a generic be first tried if it is available and the doctor does not specifically direct otherwise.

Medicare does not have such a requirement for its Part D drug component, which may be costing the government over $1 billion a year unnecessarily.

OVER THE COUNTER DRUGS

Over the counter (OTC) drugs are things you can walk into the drugstore and buy without a prescription. This includes cough syrups, cold medications, digestive remedies, and painkillers such as aspirin, acetaminophen (Tylenol), ibuprofen (Advil), and naproxen (Aleve). Some formulations of many of these include other drugs or feature higher dosages and therefore require a prescription. Others need to be purchased at the pharmacy counter because they contain pseudoephedrine. However, the pseudoephedrine formulations that must be purchased at the pharmacy are not necessarily prescription and are still considered OTC.

OTC drugs are not harmless.

Taken incorrectly, in large quantity, or in conjunction

with certain other medications, they can kill you just as dead as a massive overdose of illegal heroin. A poison expert I know considers acetaminophen to be the most dangerous drug in America because while it is generally regarded as a benign headache remedy, an overdose has the potential for serious liver damage and kidney failure. What's more, this reaction isn't immediate, so by the time the damage is recognized, it may be too late.

If your brother routinely takes *any* OTC drugs, his health care team needs to be aware of it. This includes vitamins, minerals, painkillers, homeopathics, digestive remedies, and most stuff you get at the health food store.

It is not uncommon for a drug which previously required a prescription to go OTC. This has happened in recent years with such antihistamines as Allegra and Zyrtec, as well as Prilosec and Zantac on the digestive front. Sometimes the newly-freed drug will actually cost more when this happens than when you got it from the pharmacy.

Generic versions of these medications frequently become available around the same time. They won't necessarily be cheap, either.

ANTIBIOTICS

We've all made jokes about penicillin when discovering a furry green something in the back of the fridge.

That's because we have never lived in a world that didn't have antibiotics.

The fact of the matter is that antibiotics are new kids in town, medically speaking. They didn't come along until 1928 and then only by accident, when the somewhat untidy Sir Alexander Fleming (then simply Dr. Fleming) left a culture in his lab partly uncovered when he went on vacation. He returned to find a mold had contaminated the culture—and had also killed the bacteria he was growing.

Antibiotics had the miraculous ability to cure infections, including a lot that previously might have been fatal. Who knew antibiotics would change everything so dramatically? Or that the bacterial world would fight back so aggressively, creating the kind of superbugs that make smart people never want to have to spend a night in a hospital?

These superbugs are discussed in the "Hospital World" chapter, and their resistance to conventional antibiotics has rightly scared the pants off the medical profession. The Centers for Disease Control (CDC) says that two million Americans contract disease-resistant infections annually, and 23,000 of them die from them.

In addition, antibiotics are routinely fed to animals being raised for food, so those chicken nuggets and burgers may also offer unordered and unprescribed antibiotics.

As a result of all this, a lot of people have become very self-righteous about not wanting to take antibiotics. In general, this is a good thing. Antibiotics are useless against viral infections, which includes the common cold, and if you take them when you don't need them, your body becomes accustomed to having them around and requires larger doses when you do.

However, when your seriously-ill sister needs antibiotics, this is not the time for anxiety or lectures about over-prescription.

She should take the pills, and take every single one of them even after the symptoms go away, just the way they always warn you on the label. She might want to concurrently take probiotics if she's prone to yeast infections or gastric distress, since antibiotics do not discriminate between the good bacteria that populate a normal gut to aid digestion and the bad bacteria that are causing the current infection elsewhere.

Pay attention to the label for timing of antibiotic dosage relative to food ingestion, if it's mentioned, and look it up if it isn't. This information is included in the tiny print on the flyer that may have been included with the prescription. That gets tricky, though. In addition to being filled with complex chemical lists and diagrams, those flyers are almost impossible to read without a magnifying glass. It's a lot easier to look it up online.

PAINKILLERS

Painkillers may be OTC or prescription, and both are easy to abuse. This does not mean that somebody in pain should chew on a nearby branch rather than take prescribed meds, but it does mean that everybody should pay attention where painkillers are concerned.

Caution is urged. More Americans die of prescription drug abuse than gunshot wounds or automobile accidents, and these fatalities are rising most quickly among women from 45-64.

Prescription opioids (synthetic narcotics) such as Vicodin, OxyContin, methadone, and a new painkiller called Opana (oxymorphone) need particular scrutiny. Recently some of the drugs containing hydrocodone have been reclassified by the Drug Enforcement Administration (DEA). You can learn more about specific drugs at www.dea.gov/druginfo/factsheets.shtml under Drug Info.

To combat abuse, the FDA has also recommended changes to reduce the number of refills on a prescription without revisiting the doctor. Patients would also be required to hand-carry the script to a pharmacy rather than having it delivered electronically or by phone.

Abuse of painkillers is hardly new (remember Elvis?) but general usage is up significantly. Five billion pills containing hydrocodone were dispensed to 47 million patients in 2011. That's a lot of painkillers.

People on painkillers for prolonged periods often notice that the dosage becomes ineffective and needs to be boosted for pain relief. This is called tolerance, and some recent studies seem to show that patients weaned off heavy doses of opioid painkillers actually report less pain when they're back to zero.

The flip side of this is the patient who is afraid of addiction (or has a history of addiction) and refuses to take any painkillers at all, even when she is obviously suffering. Help your sibling seek a comfortable middle ground and don't be afraid to bring up pain issues with the medical team.

Pain is an unfortunate component of a great many different types of illness, and if it's part of what your sibling is dealing with, you'll want to pay close attention, experiment with alternatives if it's safe, and see what works. There is a vast literature on pain management.

INTERACTIONS

In addition to possible problems with individual medications, all sorts of prescription and OTC drugs also interact with one another. These interactions may cause a medication to be more effective, less effective, or even life-threatening. It's a lot easier to check first than to deal with problems later. And checking is easy: Just Google the drug's name plus "interactions."

For instance, Augmentin is a commonly prescribed antibiotic. I just Googled "Augmentin interactions" and immediately learned that 69 medications are known to interact with it. In addition, the drug is countermanded in the case of certain diseases, which is why your brother's doctor ought to be familiar with his entire current history as well as the other drugs he's already taking.

If your brother is taking a number of medications prescribed by different doctors, you might want to gather them all up and take them to the local pharmacist, who will be able to alert you to potential problems or interactions. Include any vitamins or supplements in the bag when you go in.

HERBALS & HOMEOPATHICS

Many people are distrustful of prescription and OTC drugs, preferring to use herbal and homeopathic remedies. This is just fine, so long as the herbals and homeopathics are actually accomplishing what you want them to do.

In the case of major illness, however, this belief may stand between the patient and meaningful treatment. 21st Century medicine is not without its problems, but there are times when it is foolish to avoid it. (Of course, *this is not your illness.* If your sister absolutely refuses the drugs you think she should be taking, that's her decision. Dammit.)

In any case, be sure that the health care team knows about any herbals and homeopathics in current or recent use. Interactions here can be deadly. For example, a Google search of St. John's Wort drug interactions just now turned up 711 drugs known to interact with the herb, including 99 drug interactions designated as major.

One additional issue to be aware of is that you don't really know exactly what is in various supplements and nutritional aids, which are not approved or evaluated by the FDA prior to being offered for sale. It's only when folks start to suffer side-effects (or worse) that the FDA gets involved. In addition, since FDA approval is not necessary, many of these supplements may not actually contain the amount of active ingredients claimed on the bottle. Tests that pull stuff off the shelf and analyze it show wide ranges of effective dosages, only rarely coinciding with manufacturer claims. Sometimes there isn't *any* of the alleged ingredient.

Weight-loss remedies are a particularly problematic area since people who regularly battle excess weight are more likely to try anything that might help. Add "Miracle" or "Fat-burning" to the name and even more folks will get excited.

A recent study by a national network of liver specialists showed that 20 percent of drug-related liver injuries are attributable to dietary supplements. And that's just one organ.

Be careful.

IT CAN'T WORK
IF YOU DON'T TAKE IT

This seems so obvious that it shouldn't need to be stated, but a whole lot of people are prescribed medications and don't take them.

Sometimes the prescription seems too expensive and never gets filled. Or there may be unpleasant side effects. If you discover either is the case for your sister, start by talking to her doctor, who may be able to substitute a similar medication that is cheaper or has fewer side effects.

More commonly, somebody will stop taking a drug because it's invisible in a way, showing no obvious difference whether you take it or not. This is frequently the case with medications to control blood pressure or cholesterol, and it can be very dangerous.

Pay attention to what each medication is supposed to be doing, and if you don't understand its function, *ask.* It's a good idea to let the pharmacist go over any prescription when you pick it up the first time, or later if you're confused about anything.

And if your sister decides to stop taking something she has been prescribed, let the doctor's office know. Right away.

COSTS OF DRUGS

Americans spend more per person on drugs than any other country, somewhere in the neighborhood of $300 billion overall. That's a pretty pricey neighborhood.

These prices are maddeningly and irrationally inconsistent with drug prices in other developed nations, most of which have some form of national health care system. In those countries, the government can negotiate what a company will be able to charge.

Not so in the US of A.

Thanks to free spending pharmaceutical lobbies, Congress has not only forbidden Medicare to negotiate drug prices, but has also set up a labyrinth of ways for Big Pharma to charge consumers whatever the traffic will bear.

But at least there are generics, right?

Not so fast. The concept of generic drugs sounds like something that ought to be really easy, a classic example of how the free enterprise system works. It isn't.

Take the Lipitor Tale. The manufacturer of this popular cholesterol-control drug was supposed to lose its patent protection in June 2011. So they paid off a company that wanted to market a generic in a "pay-for-delay" deal. By the time it went generic in 2012, the price of Lipitor had nearly doubled since 2006. Sound a little shady? The Supreme Court has ruled that the Federal Trade Commission (FTC) can sue pharmaceutical companies for antitrust violations.

Sometimes the methodology used to get around the issuance of generic drugs can be downright sneaky. It is actually possible for manufacturers to reverse the process, going from generic to patented, with all the financial benefits that suggests.

An example in a recent series on health care costs by Elisabeth Rosenthal in *The New York Times* is the once-humble asthma inhaler, which was cheap and readily available for years, both by prescription and in lower-dosage OTC versions. Then the government banned the use of environmentally-unfriendly chlorofluorocarbon propellants in asthma inhalers.

Manufacturers not only seized on this golden opportunity to repackage and re-patent the same drugs that had always been in those inhalers, but spent half a million bucks lobbying Congress for permission.

Things heated up when scientists began to point out that inhaler propellants, sucked into the lung in relatively tiny amounts *with medication*, aren't really equivalent to, say, hair spray that billows into the atmosphere in giant fragrant clouds. Maybe an exception could be made? After all, these inhalers used very little propellant, while pleasing physicians and patients alike, and all at a very reasonable price.

Nope. Big Pharma won that battle and developed new inhaler delivery systems. Sometimes these involved genuine innovation, but even something as simple as adding a counter to an inhaler to keep track of remaining doses was enough to raise the price forty- or fifty-fold.

Rosenthal's article carried a graphic showing what $250 worth of five different medications would cost in the United States compared to foreign countries. All examples were shocking, but far and away the worst was for colchicine. This natural chemical derived from the corm of a fall-blooming crocus—one I have actually grown in my kitchen window—has been used since at least *1500 BC* to treat gout.

Colchicine was unregulated because its use predated the FDA, as well as the USA and every event in history since the tail end of the Bronze Age.

Then Big Pharma dolled it up, patented it, and marketed the new wonder drug as Colcrys. Its cost skyrocketed. Today $250 will get you 51 Colcrys pills in the US. Should you need Colcrys and find yourself in Saudi Arabia, stock up. The same sum will get you 9,158 pills.

Big Pharma exercises considerable muscle in Washington. In conjunction with other health industry organizations and manufacturers, the pharmaceutical industry spends a cool $250 million a year on lobbying, more than the defense industry.

A PRIMER ON INCESTUOUS RELATIONSHIPS: DOCTORS AND THE PHARMACEUTICAL INDUSTRY

Purveyors of drugs want to be close personal friends with dispensers of drugs, and therein lie many tales.

Even when the drugs in question are entirely legal.

If you are a Very Big Pharmaceutical Company that has just spent a few gazillion dollars developing *Epiphaneé* to combat *blortigo*, you have a strong interest in making back that investment, along with a spot of profit for yourself and your shareholders.

You will start by building up a potential customer base among ordinary people with patient potential, folks who might not even realize they have blortigo, the poor souls.

This is often accomplished through television commercials that show aging adults cavort like teenagers after taking Epiphaneé and getting their blortigo under control. The assumption is that the increasing deafness of the target audience will help them tune out the required voice-over throughout that cavorting, in which possible side-effects and warning signs are enumerated. These almost always seem to include death as well as those pesky four-hour erections.

What else can you do, Very Big Pharmaceutical Company?

Well, you can certainly suck up to doctors.

In fact, you probably already have. You may have sponsored medical research projects by influential doctors in the blortigo field or had your own esteemed physician researchers on the payroll, ready to write learned papers for journals and present statistic-packed seminars for physicians filling Continuing Education requirements. Your top-flight PR firm has been beating the self-congratulatory tom-toms in various print and online publications of the medical profession.

But most of all, you will want to make it as easy as possible for doctors to begin prescribing Epiphaneé to patients right this minute.

Not all that long ago, doctors were wooed a lot more directly, with gifts and trips and fancy dinners including spouses—the expectation being, as the late journalist Molly Ivins explained in a slightly different context, "You got to dance with them what brung you." But the industry has cracked down on its ownself, as Molly might have put it, and it's tougher now.

In just one example, if a drug company feeds a doctor, there's now a dollar limit per plate, you can't bring a posse, and you have to sit through an educational presentation. The national standard (some states are stricter) allows that dinner to cost a hundred bucks, however, which will buy you a pretty respectable meal in most parts of the country. As for the educational presentation, it will probably be given by a physician paid an honorarium by the Very Big Pharmaceutical Company.

Industry sales depend on pharma reps, the front line of pharmaceutical distribution. These sales people used to be called "detail men" back when they'd drop by my father's office to leave a bunch of samples and shoot the breeze about what was coming next from Abbott or Lilly. Now they are more likely to be twenty-something females wearing kicky dark suits with stilettos.

Their job remains the same: to leave samples and shoot the breeze with whoever in the office will listen. If that's the doctor and she gets an earful about Epiphaneé and promises to try it on her patients, all the better. Even if it's just the low-level tech who organizes the sample closet, however, that might get Epiphaneé moved front and center on an eye-level shelf.

As for you the patient, Epiphaneé ain't gonna be cheap.

But dang, it may control your blortigo!

BUCKS TO DOCS

Under a provision of the Affordable Care Act, the cozily incestuous world of doctors and drug companies is supposed to be made transparent with an interactive database available to the public. Unfortunately, the database is created and operated by Medicare and is all but impenetrable, particularly if you aren't already a whiz at databases and filters. www.cms.gov/openpayments/

Some of this information is also available through ProPublica.org. They sifted through information buried on drug company websites to compile a list of physicians and health-related institutions receiving direct payments from pharmaceutical companies. Not samples, or canvas bags, or rulers with the company logo. Cold hard cash, often for speeches given to medical personnel.

These names are now listed on its website in a searchable interactive database. Some of them bank over $20 million a year. www.projects.propublica.org/docdollars/

Another important development is beginning to change the basis on which drug sales reps are paid. Historically, their earnings have been tied to the number of prescriptions written by individual doctors. Big Pharma is backing off this model. (Many doctors are astonished to learn they can and do track this information.)

The gravy train still rolls through certain neighborhoods of the medical community. Medical specialist organizations are fair game, bound by no regulations at all. So Big Pharma and medical device providers continue to shower specialists with all manner of samples and incentives at those conventions.

DRUGS FROM ABROAD

It isn't just coke-peddling cartels and Mexican warlords who illegally import drugs into the United States any more. An untold number of otherwise respectable American citizens do the same thing every single day as they slip into a Vancouver pharmacy or a Tijuana *farmacia* or hit Send for a Canadian online order of medications.

Medications prescribed by their family physicians.

This is a matter of economics, pure and simple. The exact medication in the same manufacturer packaging may vary wildly in price from country to country. And guess which country has some of the very highest prices in the world?

Yep, it's the United States of America, where many of these medications are developed and first marketed.

When these medications are sold abroad, particularly in countries where health care is a government function, the drug manufacturer has to accept payment of what the market bears at the moment. Often that is a good deal less than what a drug costs in the US. These are, mind you, the very same drugs whether you're in Paris, Sydney, or Little Rock.

If you happen to be traveling abroad and do some advance research, you may find ways to buy drugs you use at a considerable savings in other countries. But not everybody travels internationally, so most folks turn to the internet for these international drug sales. And here is where things get a little tricky. Because guess what? There are crooks out there, selling things that look like genuine drugs but which may be poorly manufactured generics or worse.

If you choose to look abroad for the online purchase of medications, do your homework and be wary of things that look too good to be true. When you're researching, look for websites associated with long-standing brick-and-mortar retail operations.

And if you happen to be traveling in the country where your medication is made, you might consider stocking up, though not in such quantities as to get everything confiscated at

Customs.

Technically it is not legal to import any medications. A decision to break the law is, as always, up to the individual.

OFF-LABEL USE

Drugs are developed to deal with specific diseases or symptoms, but sometimes through serendipity it turns out that the medication developed to control *mediocritis* also does a pretty good job—maybe even a better job—of treating *hypocrititis*.

If this secondary result is noticed early on, it may shift the research focus altogether, particularly if *hypocrititis* is something that modern medicine hasn't quite gotten a handle on yet. But more often a drug which goes through the entire research and approval process reveals its other capabilities after it's been on the market a while, rather like a long-lost cousin who seems a little boring until he starts juggling flaming batons.

A classic example of this is the blood pressure medication Minoxidil. Men taking this oral drug to control their blood pressure began to notice an astonishing side effect: They stopped getting bald. In fact, if they hadn't been bald too long, their hair actually grew back. It seemed like a miracle and it happened right around the time when the baby boomers were first finding a touch of silver at the temples and a little more hair in the comb.

It took some maneuvering, but before all that long, you could walk into any drugstore in the land with a prescription and buy Rogaine, Minoxidil reformulated to be applied directly to the scalp. Best of all from the drug company's viewpoint, if you stopped using the medication, the benefits would also stop and the new hair would go away.

A drug grounded in vanity that you had to take for life—could it get any better? Minoxidil is now available OTC and unpatented.

Most of the time off-label treatments are a good thing. I have taken medication for an off-label use and found it a blessing.

But Big Pharma has recently gotten into a bunch of trouble for promoting off-label use too aggressively. GlaxoSmithKline paid $3 billion (yes, that's a "B") in fines in 2012 for marketing drugs for unapproved uses. And it was only one of nine companies whose fines totaled $5.5 billion that year. Perhaps most disturbing is that many of these fines were related to aggressive off-label promotion of psychiatric meds. For children.

MEMORY AND DRUGS

Some drugs affect memory in ways that are unanticipated and unwelcome. The phenomenon of "chemo brain" in cancer patients has become well known (and generally reverses over time), but many other medications can also inhibit memory. If your sibling is taking a new medication and notices a certain memory murkiness, be sure to mention it to the doctor.

The flip side is drugs designed to help retain and restore memory functions, either for dementia or as an alleged brain boost for the aging. So far none of these work very well, alas.

MEDICAL MARIJUANA

Marijuana has been on an uphill trudge toward respectability and legality since the baby boomers were kids, getting high and howling as they watched *Reefer Madness*. Lenny Bruce, who claimed not to smoke pot but used pretty much every other illegal drug and died in 1966 at 40 of a heroin overdose, once said: "Marijuana will be legal someday, because the many law students who now smoke pot will one day be Congressmen and they will legalize it to protect themselves."

That hasn't happened, but in recent years, grass roots movements (so to speak) have led to the legalization of medical marijuana by voters in twenty-three states and the District of

Columbia, as of January 2016. Most of these are in the Northeast and West, with only a couple of states from the heartland. Recreational use has also been approved in Colorado, Washington, Oregon, Alaska, and the District of Columbia.

The list of medical conditions, symptoms, and side effects for which patients have reported relief is seemingly endless. It began with nausea relief for chemo patients and appetite stimulation for HIV/AIDS patients and has continued to grow, sometimes in previously-unimaginable directions.

Perhaps the most remarkable of these is a special formulation with no hallucinogenic properties called Charlotte's Web. This has been successfully used to treat children suffering from recurrent, sometimes almost incessant, epileptic seizures.

Observing this medicinal use was one element leading to the announcement by CNN Medical Correspondent Dr. Sanjay Gupta that he believed medical marijuana should be legalized, a very public about-face.

Jokes and opinions about medical marijuana abound, with precious little in the line of cold, hard facts. Research on the use of marijuana for *anything* remains virtually nonexistent because the federal government still classifies marijuana as a Schedule I drug, a category which includes all manner of nasty things, including a bunch of opioids, heroin, LSD, peyote, and cocaine. The DEA website states: "Schedule I drugs are considered the most dangerous class of drugs with a high potential for abuse and potentially severe psychological and/or physical dependence."

One huge problem this creates in states where medical marijuana has been legalized is the direct contradiction between federal and state laws. In jurisdictions where local government disapproves of the concept of marijuana for *any* use, needy patients can have a great deal of difficulty no matter what the local law. California was the first state to legalize medical marijuana in 1996, yet local government in my home county of San Diego has actively opposed implementation of sale points ever since.

The nation appears to be at a tipping point on this issue, however. For the first time ever, national polling shows a majority of Americans favoring recreational legalization, with much of the die-hard anti-pot sentiment centered in the older population.

Your brother's doctor may be old school on this one, insisting that marijuana is a dangerous Schedule I drug that will only make his condition worse. If that's the case and your family believes otherwise, you may choose to disregard that claim.

What happens next depends on where you live.

If you are in a state with legal medical marijuana, you can probably find a doctor who will examine the patient and issue whatever legal authorization is necessary in that jurisdiction. From there, you can look for a dispensary or co-op which will help you select the strain and formulation best for the medical problem you're facing. Many of these resemble high-end chocolate emporiums, with small clusters of perfect buds on tiny plates behind a glass counter. Edible formulations that avoid smoking are available, along with a dizzying array of equipment designed to make marijuana use smoke-free. The Magic Brownie has come full circle.

Numerous Internet services also will provide overnight delivery service once you have provided the proper documentation.

If your state does not allow the use of medical marijuana, most adults have access to a young person with sufficient social contacts to obtain the medication for them. Don't be shy about asking your children or their friends for help, unless of course they work for the DEA.

ORPHAN DRUGS

Orphan drugs are just exactly what they sound like: medications for obscure afflictions that not many people have, but which are really unpleasant. These sometimes turn into made-for-TV movies, generally involving parents trying to save the life of a desperately ill child.

If an orphan drug is discovered accidentally as a property of something else altogether, even better. The company still gets all the glory. One benefit to the patient used to be that in either case, the price couldn't be too ridiculously high or Big Pharma would appear shamefully greedy.

There is, alas, a movement away from that model, and that movement gained a poster boy when a millennial hedge fund millionaire bought a company with an obscure antiparasitic drug and promptly raised its price over 5000%. Even Congress was offended by that.

Your best bet for learning about orphan drugs is a specialist in the disease or a support group of people who are dealing with it. If the disease is particularly rare, that will probably be an online group and you may be one of only four members, but if one of your motley little quartet has some information, you're way ahead of the game.

WHAT IF YOU CAN'T AFFORD A DRUG?

Some drugs are so expensive that it doesn't matter how well they work: You can't afford them.

This is particularly true of cancer drugs, which can cost up to $100,000 per dose. Insurance companies may refuse to pay for extremely expensive drugs (or other treatments), often labeling them experimental to justify the company position. Meanwhile, you've got somebody who needs help and can't afford it.

Or your situation may be less dramatic, with a patented medication that is perfect for a condition but costs several hundred bucks per month. It's not a hundred grand, but it's still more than you can afford without giving up things like food, rent, and electricity. That doesn't mean that you can't find an affordable way to get the necessary drugs. But it does require a lot more work from the patient or the patient's advocate.

Start by comparison shopping online or locally by

phone. The disparity in drug prices within a single town can be shocking, and you may find that all you need to do is transfer your prescription to a different pharmacy. Be sure to check out online ordering as well. If it's a drug that will be taken for a while or indefinitely, some insurance plans offer mail-order service with a reduced rate for a three-month supply (generally about the cost of two months' worth).

If you're still in the hole, you can also directly approach the pharmaceutical company. Many drug companies have specific information on their websites about how to obtain medication at reduced rates in cases of extreme need. Sometimes they'll even charge nothing. This largesse generates enormous good will on an individual level, as well as improved public approval at a time when Big Pharma can really use it.

A website called Needy Meds also has links to all manner of additional options for finding the help you need to get the drugs required. www.needymeds.org/ Low-income adults on Medicare may also qualify for extra help.

Certain unique situations may require a bit of creativity. One of my high school classmates was able to obtain an extremely expensive and rare drug for her husband, who was awaiting a double lung transplant. She did this by advocating aggressively and obtaining a grant from the pharmaceutical company.

What's really great about this story is that the medication kept him alive long enough to actually get the transplant, which was a success.

DRUG DISPOSAL

The days when you could flush any leftover pills or elderly aspirin down the toilet are over.

Too many fish downstream developed extra eyes or Day-Glo fins, and while you may not care what happens to those fish, it turns out that our drinking water also often contains traces of medications. Hundreds of them. This may also include bottled water not treated for pharmaceutical removal. And no, home filtration systems don't generally remove those chemicals.

Nor is the contamination limited to rivers, streams, lakes, and oceans. These things are starting to work their way down into the aquifers that supply nearly half of the nation's water.

As much as 40% of the medicine that is prescribed today is not used. This includes prescriptions that were filled but never taken (for all sorts of reasons), medications that were changed in mid-script or that caused a reaction of some sort, and medicines that have expired.

So what can you do with them?

Start by asking at the pharmacy your brother uses. They may have a good will program to collect unneeded medications, and if they don't, perhaps they can tell you where to find one in the area. Dispose My Meds lists independent community pharmacies that have such programs at www.disposemymeds.org. Some pharmacies also sell mailers you can send in for disposal.

For do-it-yourselfers, it's possible to send those old meds to the landfill if you take a few precautions. Start by mixing the medication with something that nobody will want to fish out of your trash, like used kitty litter or coffee grounds. Don't grind up the pills or open gel caps. Then put the whole mess into a sealed jar or plastic bag and toss it into the trash. Throw the empty bottle away in a separate trash bag, and be sure to remove the label or black out pertinent information about the drug and patient.

Despite all the concern about environmental contamination, the FDA recommends flushing certain particularly potent medications anyway. These are drugs with the potential to cause death or serious injury should even a small amount be ingested by a child or pet, and for the most part they're badass painkillers.

It's also a good idea to get rid of elderly supplements and OTC remedies. Vitamins lose their effectiveness over time, as do most OTC drugs. If you don't use something regularly you might not realize just how outdated it is. Take a look at everything in the medical chest for expiration dates and get rid of the old-timers.

But exercise a little common sense at the same time. You don't need to pitch *every* medication on the exact expiration date given. Actually you don't need to pitch any medication on its expiration date. Drug companies don't tell you this, but they build a little extra time into those dates. Also you should check to see if there's an expiration date on the original packaging, if you have it. That date may differ from what the pharmacy label says, since some pharmacies automatically put on an expiration date one year after the date it was filled.

An extremely successful new program through the DEA is National Prescription Take-Back Days where you can bring unneeded drugs to collection points, often local police departments. Check with your local police department to see if they participate or know of another agency that does. A recent Take-Back Day collected 324 tons of drugs in fifty states, a quantity that increases each time the program occurs.

I've done this and it was spectacularly easy. I didn't even have to get out of the car.

But flushing sure was easier.

ADDITIONAL INFORMATION

Medicare Database on Doctor Payments
www.cms.gov/openpayments/

ProPublica.org
www.projects.propublica.org/docdollars/

•••••

Ben Goldacre
Bad Pharma: How Drug Companies Mislead Doctors and Harm Patients
Faber & Faber, 2013

H. Winter Griffith
Complete Guide to Prescription and Nonprescription Drugs, 2013
Edition
Perigree, 2012

Armon Neel
Are Your Prescriptions Killing You? How to Prevent Dangerous Interactions, Avoid Deadly Side Effects, and Be Healthier with Fewer Drugs
Atria, 2013

Physicians' Desk Reference 2013
PDR Network, 2013

PDR Consumer Guide to Prescription Drugs
PDR Consumer, 2011

PDR Pocket Guide to Prescription Drugs, 10th Edition
PDR Consumer, 2013

Elisabeth Rosenthal
"The Soaring Cost of a Simple Breath"
The New York Times, October 12, 2013

Harold Silverman
The Pill Book, 15th Edition
Bantam, 2012

Pain Management

American Academy of Pain Medicine
www.painmed.org/

American Pain Society
www.americanpainsociety.org/
847.375.4715

For Grace: Empowering Women in Pain
www.forgrace.org

Pain.com: Your Pain Management Resource
www.pain.com/

US Pain Foundation
uspainfoundation.org/
800.910.2462

• • • • •

American Cancer Society
Guide to Pain Control, Revised Edition
American Cancer Society, 2004

Deborah Barrett
Paintracking: Your Personal Guide to Living Well with Chronic Pain
Prometheus Books, 2012

Barbara Bruce
Mayo Clinic Guide to Pain Relief
Mayo Clinic, 2008

Dorothy Foltz-Gray
Make Pain Disappear: Proven Strategies to Get the Relief You Need
Reader's Digest Books, 2012

Jackie Gardner-Nix and Jon Kabat-Zinn
The Mindfulness Solution to Pain: Step-by-Step Techniques for Chronic Pain Management
New Harbinger, 2009

Alpana Gowda and Karen K. Brees
The Complete Idiot's Guide to Pain Relief
Idiot Guides, 2010

Vladimir Maletic, Rakesh Jain, and Charles L. Raison
100 Questions & Answers About Chronic Pain
Jones and Bartlett, 2012

John D. Otis
Managing Chronic Pain: A Cognitive-Behavioral Therapy Approach Workbook
Oxford University Press, 2007

Donald R Tanenbaum and S. L. Roistacher
Doctor, Why Does My Face Still Ache? Getting Relief from Persistent Jaw, Ear, Tooth and Headache Pain
Gordian Knot, 2012

Melanie Thernstrom
The Pain Chronicles: Cures, Myths, Mysteries, Prayers, Diaries, Brain Scans, Healing, and the Science of Suffering
Farrar, Straus and Giroux, 2010

Craig Williamson
Pain-Free Sitting, Standing, and Walking: Alleviate Chronic Pain by Relearning Natural Movement Patterns
Shambhala, 2013

SECTION SIX:

CAREGIVING

THE WORLD OF CAREGIVING

Remember, you can sacrifice yourself—
but that won't save them.

Caregiving is one of the most gratifying of all life activities. It is also one of the most frustrating, debilitating, exasperating, and demoralizing.

How you respond to caregiving responsibilities depends a lot on who you are, what you've been doing for most of your life, what you've been doing most recently, and what you'd be doing if this situation hadn't suddenly been thrust upon you.

Equally important is the perception of what the patient is like and how long this caregiving honor/imposition is going to last.

Three weeks while your sister recovers from a knee replacement? Piece of cake.

Open-ended through radiation and chemotherapy and whatever may happen after that? A lot tougher.

Indefinitely after a brain trauma or stroke, or growing progressively worse with dementia? Moving into superhero territory, with a heavy dose of heartache.

CAREGIVING RESOURCES

The good news is that you are most assuredly not alone. According to the National Alliance for Caregiving there are 66 million (that's 66,000,000, quite a lot of zeroes) family caregivers in the United States today, and that was before you came along to swell the ranks.

This translates into a whole lot of people in the same boat, almost a third of the adult US population. This can work to your advantage in many useful ways. Your best overall resource to get started is probably the American Association of Retired People (AARP), which features an excellent Caregiving Resource Center on its website. www.aarp.org/home-family/caregiving

I also really like the AARP blog, which features links to new studies or developments in caregiving and health care, as well as most of the other issues we're looking at in this book. AARP's Family and Caregiving Expert Amy Goyer has been involved in both parental and SibCare and wrote *Juggling Life, Work, and Caregiving,* a comprehensive manual filled with useful information. If you're going to be heavily involved in caregiving, this is a great place to start.

There's also a staggering number of other caregiving books, ranging from spiritual and philosophical to how to change a catheter. Many diseases have specific caregiving volumes, most notably cancer, Alzheimer's/dementia, and brain injury/damage, a growing area.

One extremely accessible series of caregiving books comes from Care Trust Publications. *The Comfort of Home: A Complete Guide for Caregivers* is now in its fourth edition and has given rise to editions specifically devoted to Multiple Sclerosis, Stroke, Parkinson's, Alzheimer's, Chronic Lung, Chronic Heart Failure and Chronic Liver Failure.

The Comfort of Home for Stroke was right on target for an illness I had become all too familiar with and I wish I'd had it when I needed it.

You might also want to look at some of the thoughtful

pieces in *Voices of Caregiving* and *An Uncertain Inheritance: Writers on Caring for Family.* Even though it will often seem as if you are utterly adrift and apart, others have gone before and are paddling alongside you.

FAMILY CAREGIVERS

Nobody really has any idea how many family caregivers are in the United States, because people with clipboards aren't going door to door asking impertinent questions. To further complicate matters, there are many different official and unofficial definitions of what constitutes caregiving.

We also don't know the total value of family caregiving in dollars and cents, though there are some pretty staggering estimates. The Congressional Budget Office (CBO) estimated that in 2011, family caregiving for "older persons" represented $234 billion ($234,000,000,000, oh my!) The AARP Public Policy Institute had a 2009 total of $450 billion ($450,000,000,000, oh my-my-my!). The discrepancy comes down to who's included and the hourly wage used for computations: $21 by the CBO and $11.16 by the AARP. There are other differences, and the two studies don't mesh all that well, but if you have any doubt that undercompensated family caregiving represents big bucks, go back and look at those zeroes.

Family caregivers are rarely paid, though other relatives may slip them something under the table and occasionally they qualify for assistance through a governmental program or grant. Usually it's whoever is around and available. Or less unavailable.

In the past the hierarchy was clear. Children cared for parents, daughters more than sons. If you were the only daughter, your goose was cooked at birth.

Now and then siblings also cared for one another, particularly where one had never married, or was widowed. Or maybe when both were. The configuration didn't matter so much as the need, and family counted.

Not much has changed. Children still care for parents, though frequently by checkbook at a distance. Daughters still get snagged more often than sons, particularly if they have been living alone. And with increasing regularity, sisters and brothers come together in varied configurations.

What's different today is that nobody really expected to be caring for siblings. It just kind of happened.

FAMILY CAREGIVING AND THE FAMILY & MEDICAL LEAVE ACT

The Family and Medical Leave Act (FMLA) was an excellent step in the right direction, permitting an eligible employee to take up to twelve weeks of unpaid leave to recover from a serious medical condition or to care for an immediate family member—defined as a spouse, child, in-law, or domestic partner.

Siblings don't count.

SUPPORT GROUPS

When you are a caregiver, you need a lot of support yourself.

Whatever system you already have in place—family, friends, coworkers, church members, neighbors—becomes doubly important. Feel free to lean on these people, particularly if they ask what they can do. It may seem petty to say, "Come to lunch with me," but if that's what you need, it's fine. As is saying, "Stay with her so I can go to lunch."

In addition, work to cast the net a little wider. If you're caring for somebody with a specific disease, there is bound to be an online group for that, and maybe forty. Start with the website for the disease, and if you aren't satisfied with one group, move on. Somewhere online there's a format and a group just for you. If this is not a type of internet research you're comfortable with, ask somebody who is to find the group, get you set up and show you how to stay connected.

There may also be a face-to-face support group meeting in your area. This is more likely to be true for widespread afflictions like Alzheimer's and cancer, but may also be available for other medical situations depending on where you are.

The sooner you hook up with these groups, the better.

This is not just to help you feel better about the sense of loss you are experiencing, though it can certainly be useful for that. In the beginning at least, you also need a hand in figuring out what to do, and how and where to do it. After a while, you may find that you're answering questions yourself as a part of the community. Some of the best internet disease groups work that way.

This is not an either/or situation. Critical information can flow from both online and in-person types of groups, but virtual hugs lack the immediate comfort of the real thing.

In almost every situation, you'll be coming into groups already in progress. Most online groups, particularly those sponsored through well-established websites, have people dealing with every stage of the caregiving experience from fear-of-diagnosis to eulogy. This may take a little sorting out at first, but new passengers are always getting onto the train and veterans instinctively offer a hand as they climb aboard. Many lists include specialists in the field who can answer general medical questions or suggest avenues to explore.

Local in-person groups offer compadres in the trenches of local caregiving, people who have seen it all already. They know who the best local doctors are, the pros and cons of medications and treatments, what needs to be handled right this second and what can wait, and what caregiving options are available in the area, both at home and in residential facilities.

Having a live body attached to a name can be a wonderful gift. At times you will want to make a phone call and meet up for coffee, knowing that the person you're going to see will understand totally when you say, "I am going stark raving mad" or "At this rate, I'll kill her by Friday."

(You might want to take a table away from others or speak softly if you're venting these kinds of concerns in public.

Should some busybody stranger intervene, explaining that you are a caregiver won't help. And you really don't want to find Adult Protective Services knocking at your door, unless you're the one who called them.)

If you're having trouble finding some kind of live support via online connections, back off and do it the old fashioned way. Ask at the Senior Center, your church or synagogue, or even at the local Place. As in: "You're not going to put me in some *Place*."

Indeed, if the situation is really bad and family members are just getting involved at the eleventh hour, you may need to start with the Place. They will be happy to provide leads and counsel, since they know there's a good chance you'll be back later with your sibling and a big fat check.

GERIATRIC CARE MANAGERS

If you have little experience with caregiving issues and have suddenly been thrust into the forefront of a situation that seems to grow more complicated by the minute, you may want to hire a geriatric care manager.

This is particularly true if you will be caregiving at a distance.

Geriatric care managers are specialists in all aspects of care for the elderly (including the baby boomers, by definition if not self-image) and can work with you to determine your sibling's needs and the best ways to fill them locally. They can also help sort out issues if your family is at odds with one another about what to do and how to do it.

These people do not work cheap, but the expense of an initial consultation may be well worth it in the long run, particularly if you're already wrestling a few too many alligators. A bonus is that if a facility is aware that you're using a care manager, they may pay particularly good attention to your brother, since these folks are likely to steer future business their way if they approve.

Check for somebody local through the Aging Life Care Association. www.caremanager.org/

DISTANCE CAREGIVING

Distance caregiving sounds like an oxymoron. You can't exactly change a dressing at five hundred miles, after all, or provide a virtual bedpan. And you can only say "There, there" so many times over the phone before everybody starts feeling ridiculous.

For many people this isn't an issue. A Pew Research Center study showed that 37% of Americans live their entire lives in the communities where they were born.

But people ramble more than they used to, and you may have landed far from the old neighborhood. Or maybe your brother was the one whose boots just kept on walkin.' As folks get older, they tend to be well established geographically and disinclined to pull up roots because a sibling down south is sick. As for that ailing brother, he probably doesn't want to go anywhere either. Mine certainly didn't.

Of course relocation sometimes really *is* the best solution, on either a temporary or permanent basis. But even if nobody wants to move and the patient requires more care than he can provide himself, you still may be able to make things work.

Understand from the outset that you'll be facing some special challenges. A good place to start is with the Caregiver Action Network website, which features a comprehensive section on distance care. caregiveraction.org There's also a terrific booklet from the National Institute on Aging called "So Far Away: 20 Questions and Answers about Long-Distance Caregiving," available as a PDF. Like many caregiving resources, these do not always directly focus on sibling issues, but the basic rules and principles remain the same.

You'll need to be there in person to get distance caregiving set up and will also probably need to reappear at fairly regular intervals over the months and years to come. This is doubly important if there are cognitive issues involved. Somebody who's impaired or exceptionally stoic won't necessarily give you the true picture himself.

If you're using a geriatric care manager, once things are set up and seem to be running smoothly, it may be possible to simply have the care manager check in on your sibling on a biweekly or monthly basis, ideally with unscheduled drop-ins.

Critical Conditions by Martine Ehrenclou has an excellent chapter on distance care of hospital patients that can be extrapolated to other caregiving situations. Most of it is common sense, starting with show up (by phone), pay attention (take notes), and be kind (to everybody).

Perhaps some of your brother's neighbors or friends will have insight into local options, and maybe if one of them gets involved, you can get him to serve as your eyes on the ground after you leave. Talk to social workers at the hospital or rehab center or the staff at his doctors' office(s). Check online ratings for companies, facilities, or caregiver services.

Pay special attention to negative comments based on personal experience. You may not want to take the time or effort to investigate further, but as far as I'm concerned, rumors of questionable caregiving at a facility move it right to the bottom of the list. Particularly if you can't just pop in and make spot checks.

If you're going to hire somebody to come into his home, that person needs to come through a licensed agency or be carrying papers from God. This kind of care gets expensive fast, too. Yes, you can find good people for less, but you aren't going to be there to keep an eye on them. To oversee distance caregivers, you need to build in layers of protection.

Communicate regularly with the staff if he's in a facility, and bend over backwards to be charming. Be nice to everybody and learn names.

Be considerate, too. Your sibling isn't the only resident, and the staff needs to take care of everybody. Use email when you can, particularly if it's strictly informational and not time-sensitive. This allows the staff flexibility to answer your concerns when time is available.

Do speak with them when you think it's important, of course. Just don't get a reputation for being a longwinded pest who calls all the time to remind them that it's his birthday or that he'll want to watch the World Series, which starts tomorrow.

Send presents. Candy, fruit baskets, cookie assortments, potted plants, flowers. Send greeting cards and holiday cards that go up on the bulletin board and remind everybody that you're paying attention. Include minor holidays, too, so you can make yourself an ongoing presence at a surprisingly low cost.

Maintain vigilance, even if you wind up in a situation that feels very stable. That's actually when things are more likely to get so comfortable they become a little sloppy.

A DISTANCE CARE LOVE STORY

My brother desperately wanted to stay in the suburban Chicago house he had owned and been slowly renovating for twenty-some years. My sister and I agreed with his doctors that this was a really terrible idea, since his record of calling for help when needed was abysmal. But we bent over backwards to try to make it work following his first stroke on Memorial Day, even after an hour-long seizure later that year on Election Day that wiped out a lot more memory.

At that point, we knew that everybody had to face reality.

Reality for my sister and me seemed cut and dried.

We would sell his house and move him to San Diego, probably in his own apartment near me. A ten-week experiment in family cohabitation during a diagnostic summer at my sister's place in Seattle had not gone well, and I figured he'd be happier in sunshine anyway. He very grudgingly conceded that it would be necessary to move, with a marching-to-execution demeanor.

But when he visited me at Christmas—a trip I honestly expected would sell him totally on moving to a place where people surf year-round and poinsettias bloom in my yard—he hated it. Hated everything to do with Southern California, in fact, to the point of saying it was more like a fantasy than a place you'd live. (To me, of course, that has always been the point.) His desire to stay in his house in Chicago was so achingly palpable that I weakened by New Year's and told him we'd figure out a way to make it work.

He went back to a raging blizzard with a big grin on his face, and set about snow-blowing for the entire neighborhood.

I was working on the nuts-and-bolts mechanics of check-in systems and distance care when he had his second stroke a couple weeks later, the one that changed everything. A lot more memory was gone and now even he conceded that he couldn't stay alone in his house. We planned to bring him to Seattle for a brief period until I could get to Chicago, pack and ship a POD storage unit of his most treasured possessions, and find an acceptable apartment near me in San Diego.

Then we got lucky. Really, really lucky. Lifetime Movie Channel lucky.

The sister and brother who had spent six formative childhood years with my brother when he and their mom lived together twenty years earlier reappeared in our lives ... and took him in.

Indeed, it was a miracle, and one that caught us totally by surprise.

It did mean moving him several hundred miles to live with his stepdaughter, but he would still be in Illinois, and he'd always loved those kids fiercely. My sister and I made it clear from the outset that they could bail at any time and we'd bring him out to the West Coast immediately, no questions asked.

But that never happened. He spent two years sharing a rented house with his stepdaughter, then moved to an apartment by himself, looked in on daily by his stepson. After a year, he went from that apartment to assisted living, a few blocks away in the same small Midwestern town where he had by now grown quite comfortable.

I even had eyes on the ground who could watch the kids and whip my brother, a former cop, into line when necessary. His ex, with whom he'd remained on good terms, lived in town and was a police sergeant. She outranked him.

Not everybody is going to have the kind of incredible

good fortune that we did. Actually, it always felt to me like a clear instance of good karma coming back in a single lifetime, and I reminded my brother of that often. He always agreed.

So keep your options open. Sometimes life surprises you.

HIRING CAREGIVERS

At some point on the caregiving journey, it may become necessary to hire help.

This can vary from slipping a few bills to the lady next door who looks in on your sister each morning to hiring a kick-ass nursing service, and is most often a hodgepodge of makeshift solutions to an ever-changing set of problems. In the early stages of caregiving, arrangements often get cobbled together in a style reminiscent of the haphazard preschool child care arrangements many of us made not all that long ago.

The difference is that eventually our children were in school all day, while not all adult siblings who require caregiving are going to get a lot better or become more independent.

Many books and websites offer specific guidelines for hiring caregivers. Check out several and find one you're comfortable with. There's more information on this in the "Living Situations" chapter.

Here is where having a good local support group really comes in handy. If you're looking for part-time help, they may know of a good service or one to avoid. Specific names may even come up if you get really lucky.

MANIPULATION

Siblings start pushing each other's buttons at birth, and twins are at it even before that. Filed in everybody's memory banks are instincts and specific techniques for getting one's own way in a family setting. Even somebody who's extremely ill will instinctively know what is most likely to get matters moving in her direction.

If you think you're being manipulated, step aside for a

moment and take a few cleansing breaths. Then counter the manipulator by channeling a big old badass caregiver with twenty years on the job—somebody who's seen everything and takes no crap from anyone. You wouldn't want somebody like that actually caring for your own family member, but this persona is potentially useful to avoid falling into predictable and counterproductive family patterns.

Don't abuse or overuse this persona, but keep it handy.

Manipulation is not a skill diminished by illness. If you think you're being gamed, you probably are.

KEEP CURRENT

If you are in this for the long haul, you need to familiarize yourself with the disease or problem your sibling has. Once you fall into patterns of behavior and treatment and care, it may not occur to you to Google now and again to see what's going on with Wellington's Wallop.

Why bother? Well, for one thing, behaviors or symptoms which by now seem normal to you may be indicators of coming problems, which won't blindside you if you're anticipating them. Or maybe the FDA is about to approve a promising new drug.

And surely you want to be among the first to hear when the long-sought cure for Wellington's Wallop is finally announced.

Often you can follow new developments simply by signing up for regular updates from the website of the foundation for the disease in question. It's in their best interests to keep interested parties informed. That way, when you get in on the ground floor of some experimental treatment and recover fully, you'll be grateful enough to give them a boatload of money, and maybe endow a wing at the hospital.

Let them keep you informed. They'll probably solicit donations, too, but if you can't afford to help, don't feel guilty about it.

CAREGIVING CIRCLES

We discussed these in "Building a SibCare Team," because at the beginning you will have the best access to concerned people who want to help. Unfortunately, after a while people stop thinking they ought to do something and just sigh as they think about poor Jim, so limited since the weed whacker slashed his Achilles tendon.

If you've collected volunteers from the beginning, keep in touch with the ones who seemed most sincere about helping and most capable of following through. You can keep a site going indefinitely on CarePages or CaringBridge, or you can set up one of your own if you're handy that way and have the time.

In any case, keep communication channels flowing.

WHO'S CALLING THE SHOTS?

This is not your illness.

When somebody is helpless but stubborn, this is easy to forget. You want to just shake that silly fool and scare some sense into her. But it isn't only the law that's against you on this one. It's common courtesy and respect.

Respect your sibling's wishes even if they are totally ridiculous as far as you are concerned.

This does not mean that you can't feel inclined, or even obligated, to respectfully suggest doing something else that you think is a much better idea. Just know that these aren't your decisions to make. Keep in mind also that the treatment you are so blithely urging may have already destroyed your sister's immune system, sent her hair down the shower drain, and made her so haggard that you yearn to see her in size sixteen jeans again.

Try to maintain both empathy and objectivity. It's really hard to be analytical when somebody you love is suffering.

In addition, keep in mind that she is really sick. Really, *really* sick. And that when you're really sick you aren't always at your peak decision-making level.

Respecting your sibling's wishes is not inviolable, though you should need a pretty darned good reason to try to override them. If you and the other members of the caregiving team decide to countermand her wishes because there is no logical or workable solution, be prepared for unpleasantness for a while, and try to deal with it like grownups.

Ideally your sibling will have Advance Directives in place that clarify her desires. If not, and you reach a point where the patient really can't be involved in decision making, Viki Kind's *The Caregiver's Path to Compassionate Decision Making: Making Choices for Those Who Can't* is an excellent resource.

MAINTAIN PERSPECTIVE

When you are a primary or regular caregiver, it is entirely possible to be so close to the patient that you don't see changes that are immediately apparent to visitors who show up less often. This is true of physical problems: weight loss, lethargy, disinterest in appearance. It's also true of mental attitude, which can be all over the place. If changes are incremental, they're not always as easy to recognize as when they are huge or sudden and demand immediate attention.

So pay attention to what occasional visitors notice and say. These folks might pick up on something that was sneaking right past you and needs to be addressed.

Treatments of all sorts produce additional layers of up-and-down, so it can be impossible to tell what is making things better (the medication? the radiation? the chocolates?) and what is making them worse (side effects? lack of appetite? the treatments themselves?). There are adjustments, recalibrations, changes in regimen, and sometimes it seems as if nobody knows what they are doing.

Unfortunately, there will be times when probably nobody *does* know what they are doing, or what is happening medically. Despite technological advances that are astonishing, a lot of modern medicine comes down to hoping for the best and trying to fend off the worst.

CAREGIVING AND DEMENTIA

Caregiving becomes the primary issue in most instances of dementia, and about 80% of it is provided by relatives. This can be expensive and time consuming and exhausting. This topic is covered in greater detail in the chapter on "Memory Impairment."

TECHNOLOGY FOR CAREGIVERS

"There's an app for that."

Increasingly that is true for all sorts of aspects of the caregiving world. The more technologically savvy you (and your ailing sibling) are, the easier it is to find out whatever you want to know whenever you want to know it.

CAREGIVER STRESS

For family caregivers, stress is the woolly mammoth in the sickroom. Indeed, even professional caregivers can be stressed by particularly difficult patients. It's hard work.

So hard that we are devoting the entire next chapter to "Coping Strategies."

A BOOKENDED FINAL REMINDER

Remember, you can sacrifice yourself— but that won't save them.

ADDITIONAL INFORMATION

General Caregiving

AARP Caregiving Blog
blog.aarp.org/category/caregiving-2/

Aging Life Care Association
www.caremanager.org/

ARCH National Respite Network and Resource Center
www.archrespite.org

Caregiver Action Network
www.caregiveraction.org

Caring.Com
www.caring.com
866.824.8174

Family Caregiver Alliance
www.caregiver911.com

Federal Citizen Information Center
www.publications.usa.gov/

National Center on Caregiving
www.caregiver.org

National Alliance for Caregiving
www.caregiving.org/

"So Far Away: 20 Questions and Answers about Long Distance Caregiving"
www.nia.nih.gov/health/publication/so-far-away-twenty-questions-and-answers-about-long-distance-caregiving

Today's Caregiver
www.caregiver.com/

• • • • •

Alexis Abramson with Mary Ann Dunkin
The Caregiver's Survival Handbook: How to Care for Your Aging Parent Without Losing Yourself, Revised
Perigree, 2011

Diana Denholm
The Caregiving Wife's Handbook: Caring for Your Seriously Ill Husband, Caring for Yourself
Hunter House, 2012

Martine Ehrenclou
Critical Conditions: The Essential Hospital Guide to Get Your Loved One Out Alive
Lennon Grove Press, 2008

Amy Goyer
Juggling Life, Work, and Caregiving
American Bar Association, 2015

Jane Heller
You'd Better Not Die or I'll Kill You: A Caregiver's Survival Guide to Keeping You in Good Health and Good Spirits
Chronicle Books, 2012

Viki Kind
The Caregiver's Path to Compassionate Decision Making: Making Choices for Those Who Can't
Greenleaf Book Group, 2010

Joy Loverde
The Complete Eldercare Planner: Where to Start, Which Questions to Ask, and How to Find Help, Revised and Updated
Three Rivers Press, 2009

Richard P. McQuellon and Michael A. Cowan
The Art of Conversation Through Serious Illness: Lessons for Caregivers
Oxford University Press, 2010

Maria M. Meyer
The Comfort of Home: A Complete Guide for Caregivers, 3rd
Edition
CareTrust Publications, 2007

Nolo
Elder Care Agreement Legal Form with Instructions
Nolo Law for All, eForm only

Letty Cottin Pogrebin
How to be a Friend to a Friend Who's Sick
Public Affairs, 2013

Gail Sheehy
Passages in Caregiving: Turning Chaos Into Confidence
William Morrow, 2010

Tory Zellick
*The Medical Day Planner: The Guide to Help Navigate the
Medical Maze*
Victory Belt Publishing, 2012

Caregiving Circles
and Communication Networks

CarePages: Free patient websites, blogs, support and
community
www.carepages.com/

Caringbridge: Connecting Friends and Family During a Health
Event
www.caringbridge.org/

Lotsa Helping Hands
www.lotsahelpinghands.com/

Take Them a Meal: scheduling food deliveries from friends
www.takethemameal.com/

• • • • •

Cappy Capossela and Sheila Warnock
Share the Care: How to Organize a Group to Care for Someone Who is Seriously Ill (Revised and updated)
Fireside, 2004

Eric and Sharon Langshur, with Mary Beth Sammons (Founders of CarePages)
We Carry Each Other: Getting Through Life's Toughest Times
Conari Press, 2007

Cancer Caregiving and Support

Cancer*Care*
www.cancercare.org

Cancer Support Community (formerly The Wellness Community and Gilda's Club Worldwide)
cancersupportcommunity.org
888.793.9355

Help for Cancer Caregivers
www.helpforcancercaregivers.org

My Cancer Circle: Cancer Support Community for Patients and Caregivers, through Lotsa Helping Hands
www.mycancercircle.lotsahelpinghands.com

• • • • •

American Cancer Society
Cancer Caregiving A to Z: An At-Home Guide for Patients and Families
American Cancer Society, 2008

Julia A. Bucher, Peter S. Houts, and Terri Ades
American Cancer Society Complete Guide to Family Caregiving, 2nd Edition
American Cancer Society, 2011

Kathleen M. Foley, Anthony Back, Eduardo Bruera, Nessa Coyle, Matthew J. Loscalzo, John L. Shuster, Jr., Bonnie Teschendorf, and Jamie H. Von Roenn
When the Focus is on Care: Palliative Care and Cancer
American Cancer Society, 2005

Susannah L. Rose and Richard Hara
100 Questions & Answers About Caring for Family or Friends with Cancer
Jones and Bartlett Publishers, 2005

Kim Thiboldeaux and Mitch Golant
Reclaiming Your Life After Diagnosis: The Cancer Support Community Handbook
BenBella, 2012

Alzheimer's and Dementia Caregiving

Family Caregiver Alliance
www.caregiver.org/

•••••

Anne Davis Basting
Forget Memory: Creating Better Lives for People with Dementia
Johns Hopkins Press, 2009

Patricia Callone and Connie Kudlacek
The Alzheimer's Caregiving Puzzle: Putting Together the Pieces
Demos Health, 2010

Patricia R. Callone, Connie Kudlacek, Barbara C. Vasiloff, Janaan Manternach, and Roger A. Brumback
A Caregiver's Guide to Alzheimer's Disease: 300 Tips for Making Life Easier
Demos Medical Publishing, 2006

Nancy L. Maceand Peter V. Rabins
The 36 Hour Day: A Family Guide to Caring for People with Alzheimer Disease, Related Dementias, and Memory Loss, 5th Edition
Johns Hopkins Press, 2011

Maria M. Meyer and Paula Derr
The Comfort of Home for Alzheimer's Disease: A Guide for Caregivers
Care Trust Publications, 2007

Nancy Pearce
Inside Alzheimer's: How to Hear and Honor Connections with a Person Who Has Dementia
Forasson Press, 2007

Mark Warner
The Complete Guide to Alzheimer's Proofing Your Home
Purdue University Press, 2000

Laura Wayman
A Loving Approach to Dementia Care: Making Meaningful Connections with the Person Who Has Alzheimer's Disease or Other Dementia or Memory Loss
Johns Hopkins Press, 2011

Helen Buell Whitworth and James A. Whitworth
A Caregiver's Guide to Lewy Body Dementia
Demos Health, 2010

Vaughan E. James
The Alzheimer's Advisor: A Caregiver's Guide to Dealing with the Tough Legal and Practical Issues
Amacon, 2000

25 COPING STRATEGIES:

TAKING CARE OF YOURSELF

There's more to caregiving than taking physical care of your ailing sibling. A lot more. So take a breather to consider the second-most-important person in this ever-changing equation.

That would be you.

All of the caregiving books and websites emphasize the importance of taking care of yourself when you're a caregiver, and most offer very specific suggestions on how to do that. What follows here is designed to supplement those ideas.

Also don't limit yourself to what's mentioned on somebody else's list. I don't plan to list skydiving or spelunking, for instance, but if that's what relaxes you, go for it.

1. LOSE THE DENIAL

Start by being honest with yourself. You get no bonus points for pretending that everything is hunky-dory. Martyrdom is not an attractive quality.

Your entire family is on a very rocky road right now and it's silly to pretend that you're all gliding along like the Olympic Ice Dancing team. Also, even if your family's fashion of dealing with adversity consists of Carrying On, you can do whatever you want in private.

2. FIGURE OUT YOUR OWN STRESS RELIEVERS

This shouldn't be all that tricky. You've been an adult for a long time, and part of adulthood is dealing with stress. For some people, it's an omnipresent part of adulthood.

Run, jump, play. Take a walk, garden, watch sports. Knit, read, go to the movies. Bake, meditate, pray. Do some of these sound familiar? Use them as jumping-off points to figure out what works for you right now. Then take a peek back at your personal history and see if you can recall the things you did during earlier periods of extreme stress. You might come up with something you'd totally forgotten that will work perfectly right now.

Take a moment to daydream a bit and think through potentially pleasurable activities to see which ones soothe you. That's your short list. Pay attention to it.

3. SAY A LITTLE PRAYER

If you are actively involved in a faith community, you've probably been sharing your family's situation with other members of that community from the very beginning. If your sibling shares your affiliation or has another that is active, you've probably also had some participation from that community and its spiritual leaders.

But you don't need to be a Bible-thumper or a proselytizer to benefit from the calm that faith can provide.

It's perfectly all right to doubt, or to strongly doubt, or to not really believe anything at all. That doesn't mean you can't offer a message to the universe just in case anybody is listening. "God, if you're out there, we could use a little help here" is a perfectly permissible prayer under any circumstance.

Meditation or mindfulness training can also be useful.

Maybe you learned meditation forty years ago or just heard of a meditation group in town. Now is a good time to update your meditation skills or learn new ones. These are activities founded on the principles of calming the mind and soul. And if you'd feel silly doing this in public, there are all kinds of CDs, DVDs, and YouTube videos that can guide you in simple meditation techniques in absolute privacy.

4. AVOID DIFFICULT PEOPLE

At the very least, minimize their input and the time you have to spend with them.

Some difficult people are impossible to avoid, particularly if they are immediate family members, highly interactive neighbors, unsolicited religious callers, or the staff at the medical center. When you need to be with these folks, grit your teeth and take it, then break away as quickly as possible.

Those with a propensity toward histrionics are especially tough to deal with, because while you'd really like to clock them, there are usually too many witnesses.

Send somebody who is inclined to wail and rend garments and sob about unfairness to find a more appreciative audience at the grocery store.

A couple of counties over.

5. KEEP A REASONABLY STIFF UPPER LIP

This doesn't mean playing a perennial Pollyanna or being unrealistically optimistic. If you are a pessimist by nature, no sib will be surprised to find you gloomy in the face of adversity.

Still, you ought to bear in mind that your ailing sib is likely to be just as scared as you are. None of this is supposed to be happening. If you are the Department of Bucking Up Spirits, try to avoid breaking down in public. At least for a while.

6. CRY YOUR EYES OUT

It is not contradictory to simultaneously advise you to go ahead and cry.

Tears can be cathartic no matter how stoic you are. There's a physical release that comes from sobbing and you could probably use it. Tough guys are allowed to break down, be they patient or caregiver. You are, after all, in a situation that is at the very least difficult, if not downright grim.

It is even possible to get away with crying in public if you avoid eye contact. I am here to tell you that if you cry on an airplane, everybody will leave you alone.

Even if you're in a middle seat.

7. POLITE PUT-OFFS

You don't have to talk about it. Any part of it. No matter how inquisitive somebody might be.

If it's a work colleague or your nosy neighbor, you can say, "I'm dealing with a family health care problem, crisis or situation right now." Then change the subject—Can you *believe* this weather?— and excuse yourself.

Put off further inquiry with "Some other time" and if pressed, "I don't want to talk about that." You may need to repeat that last sentence a couple of times, louder each time.

Some people just can't believe you could possibly mean them.

8. LEARN TO SAY NO AND DROP SOME BALLAST

If you have ever worked as a community volunteer, you probably already have *Saying No* in your skill set, but you might be a little rusty. Drag it out and dust it off and practice in front of a mirror.

You may even find a selfish benefit here. If there were already things you don't want to do or people you don't want to see or responsibilities you desperately desire to shed, this can be a golden opportunity to clear some of this detritus out of your more recent life patterns. Make a vague promise to be back in touch when things settle down and then move on.

Every life has some elements that are routine but not really necessary, and you can safely let those slide. The world won't end if you don't keep to your customary schedule for a while. And if it does end, it won't be because you didn't get the oil changed or do laundry on Thursday.

Do what you have to, not what you think you need to.

9. DON'T BEAT YOURSELF UP

Not noticing is not a crime.

It's easy to see warning signs in retrospect, but there's no point in wasting time or energy in feeling guilty for not having acted more quickly. You're involved now, that's the important thing. You may have made some mistakes after the show got on the road, too. Fuggedaboudit.

So maybe you did screw something up, or miss a clue, or say something you now regret. If an apology is in order, swallow your pride and make it. Otherwise move on.

Mistakes wrapped in love can almost always be

corrected.

10. GIVE YOURSELF A BREAK

Every single day you need to give yourself at least one break.

These don't need to be fancy. When I was staying at my brother's house early on, as we were trying to figure out what was happening and what on earth to do next, I fell into the habit of taking a daily walk around his neighborhood. I cherished those walks, and I left the wretched cell phones behind when I went. (I had two, one a more-or-less-direct line to my sister.)

So take a walk, play tennis, or have your nails done. If you can't manage anything else, lock yourself in the bathroom for five minutes.

Don't feel the least bit guilty about treating yourself, even if it's just a fancier candy bar, or the donut you know you shouldn't have. Visit a museum or see a movie in the theater and spring for popcorn. Maybe you can't fly to Bermuda for the weekend, but you can get a cup of exotic coffee, or go to the ball game, or visit a nearby craft fair.

Set up standard personal rewards, too. There may be days when the prospect of having that one special glass of wine or bubble bath or half an hour watching trash TV is all that keeps you going. Don't deny yourself.

11. READ

Surveys of caregivers always show large percentages saying that what they miss the most is time to read.

So turn it around. Make the time and let something else slide. Even if it's only fifteen minutes a day with a magazine, that's time for you. You may also find that it gets easier to sneak in a bit of reading more often if you're working on something accessible and portable. This is not the time to start on the Russian classics.

When I'm under a lot of pressure, I like to reread things I have enjoyed in the past. These comfort reads are my literary equivalent to comfort food. I read a lot of crime fiction and many of my favorite mystery writers have produced long-running series. Over the years when I was most actively involved in my brother's care and affairs, I would binge-read my way through one favorite series, then start right in on another.

12. MAKE CHARTS AND SCHEDULES

You may have locked this all down from the beginning, but occasionally time and events move on before everything can get properly organized and integrated. If that happened in your case, take a break to be sure you're fully utilizing the resources you have available.

After a period of time, you may have a different assessment of the situation, too. Now you realize that what you need is somebody to make dinner three nights a week, not to provide transport to the doctor's office.

Start with any lists you may have made of folks with helping potential in your sibling's circle of friends, neighbors and coworkers. Figure out if somebody has a talent that you can use right now. That might simply mean somebody to be onsite for two hours while you go get a massage or a facial or lunch or a pile of library books.

If there are complicated schedules or specific needs, share them. Make sure everybody knows their assignments and obligations. Have backup systems in place for the morning when the person who's supposed to be driving the patient to chemo wakes up with a 103-degree fever and chills.

You can share this information in a wide array of media, starting with the ever-popular pen and paper. Printed schedules can be posted. Folks use dry erase and black boards, online coordination centers, calendars, notebooks and Post-its. You can put the whole business online (password-protected, please) if everybody's at the same level of computer sophistication, or work around Aunt Beth who swears she'll figure out this interwebby stuff one of these days.

13. RESPITE CARE

If you absolutely have to get out from under the

burden of caregiving—to go to Stockholm and pick up a Nobel Prize, for instance, or to go off for a weekend with your oldest girlfriends in the world, or just to go home and sleep in your own bed—some assisted living facilities offer Respite Care. This is a daily or weekly service for somebody who isn't a resident but maybe could be, and who knows?

Potential bonus: You might find out you all really like it. Even the patient.

14. AVOID MULTIPLE HEARSAY

There aren't a lot of upsides to serious illness, so it may seem silly to warn you about a particular downside which is universal, albeit particularly common to cancer. I'm going to do it anyway.

Everybody has stories about people whose medical problems were similar to your sister's and what happened to those people. I mean *everybody*, as in everybody you personally know or have ever known in your life. And the farther removed the connection (think Six Degrees of Kevin Bacon and substitute "esophageal cancer" or "lymphoma" for the actor's name) the less likely you are to receive accurate information and solid medical reporting.

Multiple medical hearsay wouldn't matter so much if the stories all had happy endings where everybody lived another thirty years and frolicked in fields of flowers. People are happy to hear those stories.

I loved being able to tell the families and friends of those newly diagnosed with brain tumors that my brother had survived an anaplastic astrocytoma (essentially a stage three malignancy) for fourteen years before his health took an unexpected but related turn. They were always grateful for a ray of positive light and I was telling the absolute truth.

Unfortunately, other people's stories are far more likely to be doomsaying accounts of Everything that Went Wrong.

You don't want to hear those stories.

So very politely cut people off. If it's somebody you see regularly, say, "I'm sorry, but I really would prefer to save your story for another time." Practice saying it in front of a mirror if necessary, then just keep repeating the same answer until the clueless one shuts up or you start to scream. Bursting into tears is also permissible at this point.

If "another time" won't work because it's somebody you almost never see but happened to run into in the grocery store, try this alternative: "Forgive me, but I really don't want to talk right now. Keep us/him/her in your thoughts and prayers."

That volleys the ball back to the person who was about to spill her family's horrible tale of malpractice, calamity, and death. An assurance of good wishes for your sibling will almost certainly follow, and you can flee as it does.

15. COMFORT FOOD

Sometimes all you really need is rice pudding, or meatloaf, or mashed potatoes, or hot cocoa. Chicken soup or a big bowl of noodles. Whatever works for you.

16. FLOWERS

Almost everybody likes flowers, even hulking he-men with Harleys parked out front. They're an inexpensive mood-brightener now found year-round in most major grocery and big box stores below the Arctic Circle.

Flowers are a great way to treat yourself to a reward that lasts for days and sometimes weeks. They're also pretty cheap if you go with what's in season. In fall, mums are everywhere, both cut and in pots. In December, pick up a bright poinsettia. In March, daffodils start showing up and by summertime, all sorts of things are likely to be blooming locally no matter where you live.

If you get something in a pot and eventually it dies, toss it with no regrets. It did its job or you wouldn't have kept it around for so long.

17. MUSIC

Listen to the music you love.

That may seem obvious, but if you're in a hushed

sickroom setting or you think you're just too busy, it's easy to forget that listening to music these days is as simple as a set of earbuds and a device that slips in your pocket. If you don't have one or know how to use it, find a young person to help you get started.

This can be particularly helpful if you and your siblings are on opposing musical planets, country-rock versus opera, say, or heavy metal versus bluegrass.

And if it isn't really possible to listen to what you want in the house, you can crank up the sound system when you're alone in the car till it blasts through to next Wednesday.

18. TV AND MOVIES

You can find pretty much anything you have ever seen or wanted to see if you look around online. Movies are often available for free or very inexpensive checkout at local libraries. The big video rental stores are mostly gone now, but vending machines dispense DVDs outside grocery stores. More live streaming options are available all the time. And don't forget dedicated cable movie channels like TCM.

Figure out something you always wanted to see and watch it. Watch all the Oscar winners through history, or every movie Steven Spielberg ever made, or all the Shock Theater horror flicks you were sometimes allowed to stay up for on childhood weekends.

If the atmosphere has been getting gloomy, comedies are a good bet, particularly ones you know you found funny before. Norman Cousins started a national health movement dedicated to the proposition of laughing oneself back to health from serious illness.

It is also now possible to binge-watch hundreds of television shows from the past and present. You might want to avoid medical shows, which may offer a little too much reality under the circumstances. But whether you want to hang out with Beaver Cleaver, Tony Soprano, or Charlie's Angels, it has never been easier to bring them home for the weekend.

19. COMPUTER GAMES

I often have some kind of game or puzzle going, and I am engaged in a profession practiced at a computer. So playing computer games to chill out has been natural and constant for me.

The term "computer games" covers a lot of territory, everything from counting ducklings for preschoolers to explosions and gruesome mutilations for gentlemen of all ages. The kind of games I like are probably different from the ones you enjoy. I gravitate toward matching games like *Bejeweled* and *Luxor* and *Candy Crush,* and I don't want to interact with other players.

Maybe your preference is *World of Warcraft* or *Call of Duty.* Or maybe you never got past *Tetris* and the solitaire that came on your computer, and you're happy that way.

It doesn't matter. Just go ahead and play it.

If you're transitioning from (or supplementing) physical playing cards and solitaire, there are programs and online sites galore for any permutation of solitaire ever devised, as well as programs allowing you to play card games that normally require other players. These are available to play either independently or online with other gamers.

20. HAVE A SPRITZ

The spirit-lifting quality of fragrance hasn't changed all that much since we were kids watching our parents put on Old Spice and Chanel No. 5. If you have a favorite fragrance now, dab on a bit occasionally or when you are feeling particularly blue.

Or you could go retro. I started thinking about the fragrances of my teen and college years and then asked for input from my Facebook friends. I got nearly two dozen different fragrance names, including a number I had forgotten about but once owned and wore.

The female fragrances that people recalled covered a lot of territory. Those with multiple mentions included White Shoulders, Jean Nate, Chantilly, Shalimar, Youth Dew, Muguet du Bois, Jungle Gardenia, and Avon's Hawaiian White

Ginger. ("Bing, bong—Avon calling.") Guys had less choice than girls back then, mostly limited to Canoe, Jade East, Hai Karate, and English Leather. ("All my men wear English Leather, or they wear nothing at all.")

You might also look into reproducing other seductive smells of childhood, though I must caution that burning leaves outdoors is against the law in many places. And don't forget incense if it once calmed you. Who knows? It could happen again.

One major caveat: If you are spending time around the patient, be sure that there isn't any current sensitivity to scent. Many medications and treatments lead to queasiness.

If your spirits are lifted but your sister throws up at the first whiff of Shalimar, at best you are playing a zero-sum game.

21. BORROW A DOG

It can be wonderfully gratifying to hang out with a reasonably well trained dog who just wants to be your friend and make you happy. Or even with a dog you don't know very well who likes to take walks or chase sticks at the park. Being able to take that dog back to somebody else's home when you're done makes it all the easier.

22. EXERCISE

I'm not going to rub anybody's nose in dreadful statistics about how much more we all ought to be exercising. You know that already. And this is not a time when you want to let any existing exercise program fall apart.

If exercise is already an important part of your life, take a bow and keep it up. If your body expects a certain amount of a certain type of behavior and doesn't get it, it could go all sulky on you. Not worth the trouble of having to fix things up later. Just keep going.

If you're in somebody else's town, you may be able to get a short-term gym membership. Or perhaps there's some exercise equipment at your sister's house already. Odds are excellent that this equipment is under a pile of boxes in a corner of the basement. But if it's there, you're ahead of the game.

If you're on the sedentary side to begin with, caregiving may make you feel sluggish and inert. A walk around the block every day is a good start to shake that feeling off.

Don't think about it. Don't talk about it. Just do it.

23. HOW DOES YOUR GARDEN GROW?

Gardening can be a really satisfying activity for relieving stress if it's something you already enjoy. If you aren't comfortable with it, or perversely pride yourself on your black thumb, skip ahead to another section.

I have been an enthusiastic amateur gardener for all my adult life. During (and since) the years when I was actively involved in my brother's care, I found a lot of comfort and relief working in my garden, which I am fortunate to be able to do for twelve months of the year in our frost-free zone.

My brother was also an avid and creative gardener before illness overtook him and neglect overtook his yard. In the beginning, our plan to move him to Southern California included a notion on my part that he'd be able—no, *eager*—to feed his long-dormant gardening instincts by helping in my own yard. The Disney forest creatures would hand us tools or ties as we needed them and carry away the weeds in ribbon-bedecked baskets. (None of it ever happened, though I do still dream of the Disney creatures.)

I grew a lot of things from seed over those years, something I hadn't done for a very long time. I planted my first full vegetable garden in twenty years. I started some things from seed that were ridiculously hard to grow and a few of them succeeded. It was a form of soothing busywork with fairly immediate gratification. I was always keeping an eye on something that rewarded me with speedy change and results.

At least that's what I realize now. Something in the process fed my need for fast and positive growth somewhere in my life.

After my brother moved to Southern Illinois, I began to buy seeds whenever I was back there, usually inexpensive ones packaged for Wal-Mart. Once I found some outdated parsnip seed in an odd little shop on the small town's dying Main Street, and I actually harvested some parsnips I grew from that seed.

Another time I planted a pack of cosmos directly into the ground, wondering if maybe it was too early but going ahead anyway. Nothing seemed to come up, and after a while I forgot about it. Sometime later, I noticed a sturdy and lacy little plant in the general area where I'd sown the seed. I began to nurture that plant, which I was pretty sure was one of my cosmos, and it thrived under the attention. It grew and grew, but never got around to blooming. By the time it was four feet high and a couple feet wide, I wondered if I'd been nurturing a particularly adaptive rogue weed.

Then my cosmos bloomed. And bloomed and bloomed and bloomed.

24. HAVE A CUPPA

Having a cup of tea to soothe yourself is an obvious coping strategy. The Brits have done it since mastodons roamed the earth. Also it's never been easier or offered more options. You can get tea harvested by monkeys if you're so inclined, and maybe even specify the breed of monkey. If your needs are simpler there are dozens of options in any grocery store. Not to mention entire tea stores and kiosks at the mall even when it isn't Christmas.

The microwave is fine for this unless you are extremely persnickety, in which case you are already brewing your tea in some more authentic and complicated way. Just make sure that after you brew that cup of tea you sit down somewhere and relax with it for at least five minutes.

25. PUT ON YOUR OWN MASK FIRST

You know how the flight attendant always instructs you to put on your own safety mask before assisting children or others around you? That's also a perfect metaphor for how you have to integrate your life into the inevitable crises, surprises, and emergencies that so often are a part of caring for any loved one anywhere.

If you're not operating at your best, nobody else will be either. Take care of yourself first. Period.

HANGING OUT WITH YOUR SIBLING(S)

It may be a long time since you and your siblings hung out together, a situation that nobody has felt any urgency to alter. Or you may get together intermittently: going fishing every summer, getting a joint cottage at the shore, attending recitals and graduations for each other's kids and grandkids, sharing significant holidays. You may even get together regularly, serve as confidantes, and automatically share triumphs and adversities.

Probably you were together in some fashion during the final illnesses of parents and stepparents.

But regardless of where your familial baseline might be, you're likely to be spending a lot more time with each other now. What on earth will you do with that time?

SOME GOOD NEWS FIRST

This is likely to be a lot more fun than hanging out with your parents, which you may have experienced at some length during their final years.

With your parents, you usually have to do what *they* want. Their music, their movies, their food preferences.

But with your siblings you have a rich history of hanging out. It's what kids do and what you did, particularly back in the days when there was one black-and-white television and one black rotary dial phone per household, and you rode your bike for miles in any direction, and you improvised toys out of materials that have long since gone on various banned and hazmat lists.

So you're not nine any more, and the treehouse is long gone. Or maybe you never did get it, even though your dad kept saying, "Some day." The dollhouse is probably also long gone, along with the *Monopoly* and *Clue* and *Careers* board games. The four-year-old running amok in the next room is not your little sister, but your sibling's granddaughter. And let's hope, if she's running amok, that she's not *your* granddaughter.

SO WHERE DO YOU START?

Find common ground.

You may already be way past this, but if the family connections are a little rusty, it generally can't hurt to look backward. It's nice if you had a picture book childhood, but a lot of us didn't. These waters can get muddy or rocky or both.

So make an effort to identify childhood's good memories, even if they were pretty sparse. As for the less-happy times, you might also try to recall bonding moments within that framework, things that brought you closer together or perhaps events and experiences that you see now in a different light.

This is not the same as living in the past. It allows the past to serve as a bridge to bring you closer together now.

USE PROPS

If you're breaking the ice on a long-frosty relationship, props can help. Even if everybody is already pretty thoroughly thawed *and* also rather fried, they can just be fun. Comic relief is your friend.

Were there particular games or toys you played with as kids? The originals may still be around if there's a packrat in the family, and if not, you can probably find them on eBay. With a little perseverance you can probably even get the actual edition of board games that you played when you were kids. With original pieces. (If you need too much authenticity, I must warn you, this can start to get pricey.)

For instance, my family had a lot of building toys that just aren't around much in this Playskool/Fisher-Price world. We had big red cardboard bricks and little tiny red interlocking plastic bricks and millions of Tinkertoys and Lincoln Logs. I just looked them all up on eBay and found every one, in the editions we used. For the record, there were 1200 Vintage Monopoly games listed, and 250 Vintage Lincoln logs. I also saw the edition of *Careers* that we used to play, the one that was actually less sexist than later editions where career choices were things like Stewardess, Teacher, Nurse, and SuperMom.

There might also be some item of particular significance to your family, and this could be absolutely anything from a rusty manual push mower to your parents' collection of matchbooks and cocktail napkins. Was there was something you loved and your brother hated or vice versa? You might look for some of these items online, too.

A really nice picture of that mower (or one sufficiently like it) will probably suffice, however, so you won't need to crowd the sickroom.

If sports was the big deal in your family, tread lightly. Your brother might once have broken several local track records, but if he is now using a walker and having considerable difficulty with it, remembering those times may be more painful than therapeutic.

CAN'T WE ALL JUST GET ALONG?

Seek neutral ground if there are personality clashes or political or religious differences that threaten to get in the way. Look to sports, books, TV, audio books, or movies on DVD. What kind of small talk do you make in your regular life? Will it work here?

If relationships are crusty, make technology work for you. Make it work for you in any case via whatever your family's preferred methods of communication might be: text, email, Skype, streaming DVD, tablet, iPad, etc., etc. If your family's back in the Technological Dark Ages, now is not the time to drag them kicking and screaming into the New Digital World. That goes double if the one in the Dark Ages is also the patient.

Also now is probably not a good time to download a new operating system, particularly on your sister's ailing computer. If something is busted, get it fixed, but keep matters simple and in perspective. Don't make anything so digitized or so complicated that the rest of the family can't comfortably use it.

The exception is when there's a genuine Luddite, and usually you can identify these people pretty easily because they are proud to tell you in some detail how nicely they manage without smartphones and tablets and TVs that hang on the wall. In fact, they are likely to go on until you'd like to throttle them. If you should be the Luddite, I apologize. Though it's true.

Respect the patient. This is not your illness. This is not your rate of recuperation. This is not your party. Let the patient call the shots unless she is absolutely unreasonable and unrealistic and uncooperative, in which case you'll be in the next room anyway, beating your head against the wall.

KEEP THE SOUND TRACK PLAYING

Songs have associations, and you can use these to everybody's advantage. Some of this strategy is forehead-slappingly obvious: Play music that makes you feel good. This of course is highly individual but in general, soft music is soothing, rock energizing and country/western often useful when you want to feel sorry for yourself.

Whatever music works for your sibling, *use it*. And remember, too, that what works for one of you might not work at all for others. You are welcome to maintain a parallel sound track if you like. That's what earbuds and earphones are for.

Please don't try to convert an ailing sib to some new form of music. As they age, most folks have their preferences set pretty well and may, in fact, be losing their hearing. (This is not something boomers are acknowledging just yet, though it needs to be said pretty loudly in many cases.) So don't think you're going to convert a Springsteen man into an opera lover, or vice versa. It ain't gonna happen and the process of confirming that won't be fun for anybody.

However, if your sib loves Metallica and that music

makes you want to run screaming from the room, by all means run screaming from the room. A really good set of noise-cancelling headphones will also be useful.

Never underestimate the power of music to change or improve a mood.

JIGSAWS AND OTHER PUZZLES

Jigsaw puzzles are often found in locations where people spend a lot of time together in unfamiliar circumstances: jury lounges, summer cottages, rental properties at the shore or lake or mountains, waiting rooms, rec centers, cruise ships, family reunions, and sickrooms.

There are lots of reasons for this. One undeniable advantage to having a puzzle in progress on a card table or other unused flat surface is flexibility. People can work on it at their own speeds on their own schedules in various combinations or alone.

It may be that all but one person hates jigsaws—my own daughter says she never understood why anybody would take a perfectly good picture and cut it up—but that's no reason not to set one up anyway. A jigsaw-in-progress can also be an icebreaker with guests during difficult visits.

Sudoku and word search and crossword books are useful for people with limited current mobility, keeping the brain charged while other body parts heal. For the caregiver or visitor, they can also be therapeutic.

Computer games and games you can play on phones don't have as much potential for shared experience, but they're something an individual can withdraw into for short or long periods.

The really great thing about all of these is that when you're done with one, it's so easy to start another.

NOSTALGIA MEDIA

There are endless opportunities to recreate happier

times through nostalgia media. Program special music on an iPod or have somebody do it for you. This is the kind of thing that works very well as an assignment for somebody who says, "If I can help in any way..."

If there were shows you all watched together as kids, you may get a kick out of seeing them again decades later. *The Mickey Mouse Club,* for instance, might be just the ticket for somebody who always adored Annette. Maybe The Three Stooges seem a little dumb now, or maybe they're as funny as ever. It doesn't matter. The shared experience is what counts. (For the record, *Have Gun, Will Travel* holds up beautifully, though its sense of Western geography is a little problematic.)

If the only thing that your brother wants to watch is Rambo I-II-III-IV-V, let him. You can put on noise-canceling headphones or leave the room.

FIELD TRIPS

You should constantly give yourself small rewards for the services you extend to your sibling and family. One very sneaky and perfectly legitimate way to redeem those rewards is to pamper yourself and your sibling at the same time. What you are able to do will depend on the current state of your sister's health, but you can be creative.

Get manicures or take a walk on the beach. Catch a senior-discount matinee at the movie theater—and buy the three-gallon popcorn drenched in thirty-weight if you love it. Or feel free to smuggle in your own food if there are dietary concerns or limitations.

Take your brother to the ball game. Take your sister to the art museum. Or bowling. Or to the hair dresser. Or to whatever fool thing she likes to do, whether you enjoy it or not.

The object here is to make either or both of you feel better. If one of you is cheered, that can only have a salutary effect on the one who still feels pretty crappy. Or maybe you'll get lucky and come home from your field trip dancing like the Jets and the Sharks in *West Side Story.*

HOLIDAYS

Major illness changes everything, including holidays. It goes from "Do we have to get the tree out this Christmas?" to "Will we ever have Christmas together again?"

Just like that.

Holidays can be rough when you're dealing with serious illness. The temptation is to keep everything as it always has been, but often that doesn't make sense. This is particularly true if the ailing sibling is usually actively involved in the customary festivities.

If your sick sib always hosts a holiday dinner or celebration, make adjustments or change venues, and be matter-of-fact about it. It is not necessary to do everything the way you usually do. In fact, it's probably a good idea not to, since folks may not have the energy.

Adapt. Adjust. Save the parts that everybody agrees are indispensable and let go of some of the other trappings that are more pro forma than necessary.

One good approach is to maintain the customary holiday framework but scale way back. You don't necessarily require three dressings and five kinds of pie at Thanksgiving. In fact, you can get a perfectly acceptable, fully-prepared dinner and make only those side dishes that everybody truly believes are essential. The pumpkin cheesecake, for instance, or Aunt Ellen's legendary cranberry relish. The goal is familial camaraderie despite tough times, not a five-star Michelin rating.

Make some dish from childhood that nobody's had for years, or at least try to recreate it. You might even make something everybody hated just to see if it's still awful, and if it is, you can feed it to the dog or put it down the disposal. (I am thinking here of my Aunt Dotty's baked oysters, from her girlhood on the Jersey shore.)

Repeat after me: There is no dishonor in purchasing an entire prepared meal.

Lots of people do it anyway, which is why it's so easy

to get a roasted turkey or a HoneyBaked ham and all the appropriate trimmings and side dishes around any major holiday. It will save a huge amount of work, provide leftovers, and allow everybody to make (cursory) comments about either (a) how much better Mom's turkey always was, or (b) why didn't we think of this years ago?

Or you can all go out for dinner.

While it may seem like a nice idea to fix all the sick sibling's favorite foods, there's an excellent chance that the patient doesn't have much appetite anyway. So keep it simple and concentrate on good spirits rather than haute cuisine.

This does not mean, of course, to skip the wine or eggnog if that's part of the normal gathering. Folks may want alcohol even more under current circumstances. If the patient can't drink, that doesn't mean everybody else has to abstain, unless the patient is a continual whiner, in which case you have bigger problems and might just as well take that wine bottle into another room all by yourself.

Holidays can also be an opportunity to look back on shared experiences of the past.

The time Barb's elaborate Cinderella costume got drenched in a trick-or-treat downpour. The year the Easter Egg Roll was snowed out. The Christmas when Susan got a puppy and the twins got two-wheeler bikes.

Maybe your family had a special Christmas activity like cutting snowflakes out of tissue paper or stringing popcorn and cranberries. Try doing it again. Maybe you always talked about stringing popcorn and cranberries, year after year, and never did it. Give it a shot now. Make the kind of cookies that your Grandma always baked, and don't worry if they don't turn out the way hers did. Concentrate on the process, and ignore the results if you choose.

Break out the photo albums if you have them and look at all the holiday pictures from when you were kids. If there's a family techno wizard, maybe that person can digitize the highlights for a family DVD or photo book. Talk and laugh about the crazy and funny things that did or didn't happen around holidays and celebrations—dipsomaniac Uncle Ralph passing out in the mashed potatoes, Great-Aunt Edna launching her customary endless Christmas tale about being snowbound as a girl, cousin Rachel hoarding her Hanukkah chocolate coins.

Whatever there was in your shared history, dig it out and revisit it. Looking back can be a lot more satisfying and comforting than looking ahead in a period when the future is uncertain.

If looking back is horribly painful, then perhaps now is the time to acknowledge that [fill in your own family horror story here] ruined such-and-such holiday. We used to have particularly tense, alcohol-fueled Thanksgiving family dinners, and one year when I was in college, I wrote a five-act playlet called "Trauma Round the Turkey" to send to my cousin who was at the Air Force Academy and didn't have leave. If memory serves, the entirety of Act III was my grandmother saying grace.

Maybe after all these years you can laugh about some of these things, or maybe everybody just needs to have the air cleared.

PETS

Pets for the seriously ill can be a great virtue or a gargantuan pain. If your sister already has a couple of dogs, somebody needs to pay attention to them. Do they need/expect to be walked four times a day? Taken to the dog park? Brushed four hundred times each morning with a special tortoiseshell brush?

When somebody is in the hospital, pets are very aware from everybody's vibes that things are seriously amiss, but have no way to grasp or understand the particulars. Their own vibes are likely to be in overdrive as well, particularly if the last time they saw their master he was unconscious on a gurney going out the door with a lot of strangers.

Is there a neighbor who could take the dog in temporarily, or stop by to feed the cat and empty the litter box? It's a shame to board animals unnecessarily, but sometimes there isn't a choice.

Keep in mind that the relationships between pets and owners who otherwise live alone are often intense and meaningful in the most obvious codependent style. Separation is rough on all parties, and the ones with four legs may act out in societally-frowned-upon ways. If you find turds where there aren't supposed to be any, this may be what's happening. Try to find it in your heart to forgive, even if you already didn't like the pet. It wasn't the dog who gave his master cardiac arrest, and he's as worried as you are.

Getting a new pet for a sick person is a spectacularly bad idea. This is true even if you are absolutely certain that person is getting well and the recovery will be speedy.

Whether or not you say it out loud, you definitely need to think about contingency plans if your sibling is unable to care for any pet at some point. Are *you* prepared to take in that puppy, kitten, iguana, or parrot? I didn't think so. (Note: Parrots can live into their seventies, well past human Medicare age.)

TRAVEL

There are a lot of variables here, and the biggest and most important one is the actual state of the patient's current health.

In some cases, finances and relative mobility will allow for travel, maybe even some fairly serious travel. With medical permission and somebody along who knows exactly what's happening (that sounds suspiciously like you, the one who's actually reading this book), you can do a lot of traveling.

It probably isn't a good idea to take somebody with a compromised immune system into Third World jungles, even if you can afford to bring a doctor along. But most of the United States, Canada, or Europe is entirely reasonable, as well as almost any country that your family originally came from, no matter where it might be.

Do your homework. A number of excellent resources at the end of this chapter will guide you through the necessary processes and checklists. Don't bite off more than is reasonable, and keep alternatives in mind. Find out about cancellation policies when you're making reservations. Get travel insurance.

If you're traveling abroad, know exactly where you are going to be and when. Find out where the US Embassies are and what kind of medical treatment is available to foreigners. Check on what your sibling's health insurance covers where.

Make sure you have more than enough of all your sibling's current medications and carry prescriptions in case anybody bothers you at Customs. Pack a spare pair of glasses for everybody.

Think through the amount of equipment necessary and how you intend to manage it. A friend who accidentally ended up with an enormous suitcase discovered it was just the right size for her mother's commode. Yes, that's how you need to be thinking. Things that will be very hard to find if you don't bring your own along.

You can get a cane anywhere, however, though it may say Souvenir of Sorrento on it.

TRAVEL INSURANCE

Travel insurance is essential.

In some cases, it's offered automatically with special tours or cruises, and if it isn't, seek out an agent who handles it. This is not the life insurance they used to sell in machines at airports in case your plane crashed. It's what will return your investment to you if you need to cancel at the last minute or bail midway through the trip.

And it can sometimes do even more than that. A friend who fell and broke her pelvis in Washington, D.C., flew home first class to San Francisco the next day with a nurse in the seat beside her. She was in excruciating pain, but it was all covered. And then she was home.

MAKE REALISTIC TRAVEL PLANS

This is not the best time to set out to visit all fifty states, unless you're already well into the forties and have checked off Alaska and Hawaii.

Maybe what you'd really like to do is go back to some place you visited when you were young and have good memories about. The lake, the cottage, whatever. If the place your family used to go is totally gone, well, that's a bonding experience, too. You can either try to find something similar or do something altogether different and wild.

Think about local possibilities. A lot of times you don't go to places that are nearby because they're, well, nearby. You figure you can catch them some other time, or maybe take out-of-town company. Except then visitors don't come, or you end up doing something else. Most people have a surprising number of interesting resources nearby that they've never visited. I can think of half a dozen in my own area, which is pretty embarrassing. It is definitely time to visit the Surf Museum.

Just keep in mind that the sicker and less mobile the patient is, the more cumbersome any travel becomes, including getting to the doctor's office.

WHEN YOUR SIBLING TRAVELS ALONE

Set up as much in advance as you possibly can when your sibling is traveling alone. You may or may not have cooperation from the traveler, but it's important.

If wheelchairs are necessary and your sister doesn't have her own, make sure that the airline knows you'll be needing one on both ends of her trip. This will change the pattern somewhat at security screenings, and may even move you to the head of a line. If the flight serves food and she needs a kosher meal, order it.

You can get a letter from her doctor that allows you to accompany her through security to the gate and to stay there until she's safely on the plane. Feel free to take advantage of advance seating and talk to the people at the gate about her special needs. When she arrives at her destination, her daughter can pick her up at the gate using exactly the same kind of doctor's letter.

Use direct flights or routes as much as possible.

If any kind of mental confusion is part of the current picture, do all of this and then also spend time brainstorming everything that might possibly get screwed up. Cover as many contingencies as you can.

Also keep in mind that at the other end, she won't be in the familiarity of home. She'll be a visitor in somebody's home or a guest at a hotel, either of which is full of social and physical landmines.

BUCKET LISTS

I'm not a big fan of Bucket Lists, since they strike me as arbitrary and fraught with potential problems. The biggest of those problems is that you set yourself up for a feeling of failure if you don't manage everything. What you should be striving for instead is a sense of conquest and accomplishment from doing something that you always wanted to do.

Ask this question: Is this a motivator or an impossible dream? Can't it just be something fun to do? Don't set anything up as success vs. failure because the stakes are too high. Be realistic yet adventuresome.

It may be too late for the Expanded Bucket List that included climbing Mount Everest and learning Chinese, but if you pare it down to something manageable, it can be fun. A Mini-Bucket List of movies to see. Sports classics: games to watch again. Games to watch *now*. Meals to repeat. Places nearby to camp. Museums in the area.

Having an outsider's eye can help here. Just don't get too ambitious.

POLITICS AND RELIGION

Nothing will mess up a civil relationship or discussion faster than the injection of contrary political or religious views. You and your sibling and the rest of the family are already stressed by illness and uncertainty. You don't need to be fighting at the same time.

Where politics is concerned, agree to disagree and let it go at that.

If there's an election coming up and your sib customarily votes, make sure that there's an opportunity to send in an absentee ballot. You may also provide chauffeur service to the polls, or arrange for somebody else to do it.

This is the honorable way to handle an election even if you abhor everything your brother believes in and have been deleting his vitriolic political emails unread for years. Grit your teeth and make sure you get to your own polling place, to at least cancel out each other's votes.

Religion is even more personal.

If your family is all on the same spiritual wavelength, you have nothing to worry about here and you will probably all find comfort and solace in your shared faith and faith community.

If you differ on fundamental religious issues, however, this is not the time to impose your beliefs on a sibling who is a captive audience. You may think you're getting through, but it's more likely that your sister isn't so much receptive as simply too weak to argue.

If your sibling has a pastor/priest/rabbi/guru and wants that person around, then you should do your best to see that it happens as often as all parties are available and willing. Do not tell her it's a lot of hooey, or bring in spiritual advisors she isn't interested in seeing under the guise of doing what is right for the eternal sanctity of her soul.

This is the proper thing to do even if you are terrified that your sister is going to go to hell for not following the spiritual road you consider correct.

EVERY PICTURE TELLS A STORY

Get out the family photo album.

Track it down if you have to, as well as other pictures in boxes that came from Grandma's when she went into assisted living, or the trunk in the attic, or wherever. If you don't have an album, you've probably got pictures lying around somewhere. Get them out. Talk about the pictures, and the history. Laugh whenever you can.

If somebody is computer-savvy, there are all kinds of possibilities for scanning old pictures and creating online and print albums and collages.

When you come across fun photos that were long forgotten, put them in small frames and set those up where everybody can see them. If there's a pile of fun pictures, switch them out every week or so. Frames are cheap and readily available.

This can also be done electronically in digital photo frames

THE SHIFTING SANDS OF MEMORY

Remember that your memories are not necessarily the same as the ones your siblings have. Any time families get together and discuss the past, it's likely there will be spirited disagreement about what happened when, how, and to whom.

A lot of family history is like *Rashomon,* where everybody remembers things differently but is absolutely certain that theirs is the only correct recollection.

Is it really worth fighting about? You're probably better off agreeing to disagree. This is true even when you are certain that you are absolutely right.

THE DIFFICULT ONE

What if the ailing sibling is also the difficult one?

There's no getting around it. A lot of families have a difficult sibling. There are thousands of different ways in which they can be difficult, but it's not exactly unusual. Just a fact of life that most families learn to work around in their own fashion.

Tempting though it may be, this is not the time for payback. If the sick sib is the one who made your life a living hell or abused you, you are not obligated to involve yourself in any way, of course. But if it's more a question of irritating personality traits, maybe you can ignore them for a while.

No need to be a saint, however. If somebody who's always been a jackass is behaving like a jackass, you certainly may point it out.

To the jackass. In person.

IT'S THE LITTLE THINGS...

Gestures count.

Sometimes the gestures that really count are ones that bring back memories of being cared for during childhood illness. Did Mom sort little bits of food into the segments of a muffin tin to make them look more interesting and enticing? Put green grapes into red Jell-O? Make a special macaroni and cheese? (Yes, I'm talking about Kraft dinner with hot dog chunks.)

A lot of this may seem contrary to the way we are supposed to be eating now, but if somebody has no appetite and you can get some calories into her with a hideous reminder of childhood, then go with the hideous reminder. Nobody says *you* have to eat the Jell-O.

If the sib is far away (or local but you can't get by regularly) then send cards or postcards or encouraging emails. Funny is good. Inspirational is best suited to those you know will appreciate it. So is very dark humor.

And remember to be upbeat but not unrealistic. You shouldn't suggest somebody will be bouncing out of bed in a day or two if she is two weeks into six months of debilitating chemo, but do aim for a spot of cheer. Too much sorrow about illness can make a sick person start to wonder if things are even worse than they believed.

A single flower on a tray or in a small vase is always nice, whether the patient is male or female.

Live in the moment.

Additional Travel Information

Making Life Easier
www.makinglifeeasier.com

PALS Patient Airlift Services
www.palservices.org/
888.818.1231

• • •

Sue Maris Allen and Barbara Ramnaraine
Wheeling & Dealing: A Guidebook for Travelers with Disabilities
Seaboard Press, 2008

Stephen Ashley
Walt Disney World with Disabilities
Ball Media Innovations, 2008

Candy Harrington
22 Accessible Road Trips: Driving Vacations for Wheelers and Slow Walkers
Demos Health, 2012

Candy Harrington
101 Accessible Vacations: Vacation Ideas for Wheelers and Slow Walkers
Demos Health, 2007

Candy Harrington
Barrier-Free Travel: A Nuts and Bolts Guide for Wheelers and Slow Walkers, 3rd Edition
Demos Health, 2009

Andrea & Craig Kennedy
Access Anything: I Can Do That!—Adventuring with Disabilities
Outskirts Press, 2007

Rick Steves
Rick Steves' Easy Access Europe: A Guide for Travelers with Limited Mobility
Avalon Travel, 2006

SECTION SEVEN:

LIFESTYLE ADAPTATION

LIVING SITUATIONS

Most folks intend to spend the rest of their lives in their current home and die peacefully in their own beds at the age of 97. This is not always a reasonable expectation.

At some point it may become necessary to make alternative living arrangements for your sibling, particularly in the case of somebody who has been living alone and is suddenly very ill or incapacitated.

This will almost never be easy, appreciated, or fun. But there are ways to make it less painful, and some intermediate steps that may buy more independent time. Judicious use of options discussed in the chapter on "Home Modifications and Assistive Technology" might mean the difference between staying in place or needing to move. If you are able to supplement these changes with an appropriate form of check-in and reporting system, all the better.

THE PANIC BUTTON

"I've fallen and I can't get up."

We've all heard the commercial. We've all mocked the commercial. We were once incredibly young and cool.

Now that panic button can be a darned good idea.

The toughest part may be getting your sibling to agree to it, or to use it when necessary. The few, the proud, the stubborn—folks like my brother who never got around to calling for help, no matter how much he needed it.

But if you're working with somebody willing to compromise to maintain independence, this simple technology can be a wondrous thing. Your sister can wear something on her wrist or around her neck that she can punch once and know that help will come. More sophisticated versions can be programmed to call in on their own in case of a fall or prolonged shaking consistent with a seizure.

NEIGHBORHOOD WATCH

This is the simplest and easiest way to keep track of somebody with ongoing health problems who wants to keep living alone. I first saw this system in action when visiting my boyfriend's grandmother in Florida while in college: Residents turned a placard on the door each morning to show that they were alive and not in need of immediate assistance.

One or more neighbors will need to cooperate to make this work. Once you find a willing assistant, figure out the easiest system for both parties and roll with it. This may be as simple as your sister opening the curtains or pulling up the shade on a specific window each morning and reversing the process at night. Maybe there's a hook on your brother's porch where he can hang a ball cap when he gets up and bring it in again at night. Or a potted geranium that your sister can set out on a summer morn and bring in when the fireflies come out.

The system isn't foolproof and it may take a while to become a habit. But if somebody forgets or oversleeps, a call from the neighbor can confirm that everything is okay. If that call goes unanswered, set up a system for what comes next. If the neighbor is willing and has a key, that next step might be sticking a head in the back door and calling, "Hello?"

Keep in mind that this responsibility is an imposition when assumed by a neighbor, who is likely to have plenty of other things going on in the course of his life. I gave a key to my brother's next door neighbor when he lived alone briefly between strokes, but I always told her that if she thought anything was seriously wrong, to just back out the door and call

911.

For my super-patriot brother, I worked out a magnificent system where he'd put out the US flag each morning and bring it in again at sunset. Unfortunately, he had another stroke before we could get that into play. Also it was snowing pretty much nonstop and the bracket for the flag wasn't visible to the neighbor who'd be doing the watching.

But it was a brilliant idea, if I do say so myself.

PHONE OR COMPUTER CHECK-IN

This one is also easy, with numerous variants.

If there's somebody in the family who's willing to call each day at about the same time, that's an ideal situation.

My sister did this for years when my brother was living—by his own preference—half a continent away from both of us. She called every morning, usually from her car on the way to her veterinary clinic. By the time she arrived, she'd determine that he sounded okay and each could share a bit about their current lives. If something seemed amiss or confusing, she would let me know and we'd contact his local caregivers.

The check-in call doesn't need to last long, though if you enjoy speaking with one another, it can actually be a gift and benefit in both directions. You should have a backup in case you get no answer and aren't aware of appointments or problems that might explain a failure to respond. A friendly neighbor is the best option here, preferably one with a key. If that isn't feasible or the neighbor isn't answering, it's entirely appropriate to call the local police.

Numerous services and companies offer robo-calling for daily check-ins. This is the same annoying concept that reminds you of medical appointments and to vote for the people's choice for Congress. Most of these require an actual person to answer the phone. If the call kicks over to voicemail or a message machine, the machine keeps calling till it's picked up, and if that doesn't appear to be happening, the service will follow pre-arranged next steps. This may mean calling you, a neighbor, or 911.

If your sister is computer savvy, you may arrange to have her send an email to you each morning, a system that worked beautifully for my stepmother and her sister. If she's really savvy, you can opt to Skype or Facetime so you can actually see for yourself that she's okay. The only problem with visuals might be if she's feeling unattractive and doesn't want to be seen.

Illness will do that to you.

YANA – YOU ARE NOT ALONE

My local police department operates a wonderful personalized program through its Senior Volunteer Patrol. Seniors living alone may register for daily phone calls Tuesday through Saturday from a member of the patrol, also comprised of seniors. On Mondays, the Senior Patrol visits each participant to check in person on well-being. Records are kept of all calls and visits.

Couldn't be simpler, and both patrol members and participants love it.

The local senior center may be aware of such a program in your brother's area. Maybe you can even talk them into starting one.

MEALS ON WHEELS

Meals on Wheels operates in fifty states providing meal service to seniors, in this case defined as people over sixty.

Started to feed British servicemen in 1940, Meals on Wheels delivered its first meals in baby carriages pushed by nurses. Sixty years ago, the teenaged program jumped the pond. Today over 5,000 local organizations deliver a million meals a day. You can find the nearest participating group at www.mowaa.org.

The organization's stated goal is to have no senior go hungry. Volunteers deliver once a day to those who are registered. Some recipients pay and others are subsidized; check with your local organization for particulars.

The value here is in knowing that one or two meals will be brought to your sister's home each day, so that she doesn't need to do grocery shopping or cooking or cleanup. An additional bonus is that somebody will be ringing the doorbell six days a week (Sunday meals are delivered on Saturday), thus providing additional eyes on the ground to see that she is all right.

SOMEBODY WHO COMES IN

This is a common transitional step, the introduction of outside caregivers scheduled on a regular basis to visit your brother and assist with minor medical issues, various household chores, appointment transportation, and shopping.

Outside help may come from government Social Services on a state or local level. This generally requires a Needs Assessment to determine eligibility and independence levels. Since a lot of material comes out of interviewing the patient, somebody who wants to seem more independent than he really is might, well . . . fib a bit. My brother never came close to a qualifying score, and believe me, he should have.

You might be able to arrange for the somebody-who-comes-in to be an informal caregiver from family, community or church. On a short-term basis, friends sometimes set up networks such as those discussed in the chapter on "Caregiving."

Or you may need to hire somebody, which is not a reality that anybody is likely to be happy about. It involves whole different levels of business and personal complications, expense, and supervision.

How long this stage lasts is dependent on the nature of your sibling's medical problems, the likelihood of additional deterioration, and how well everybody is adjusting to the new family normal. If somebody is impaired but stable after a stroke, for instance, it can go on for quite a while and possibly forever.

However, because this kind of system *is* transitional, it

often opens up a lot of the grievances associated with a need for increased supervision. Getting these on the table won't be pleasant, but may be necessary since the stages that follow will be even more problematic.

ADULT DAY CARE

Adult day care desperately needs a better name, something like Jeff or Betsy.

It sounds just awful as it is, like some kind of preschool program except that everybody's 85 and uses a walker. If the service you are considering calls itself something else—*anything* else—for heaven's sake, refer to it that way, and say it a dozen times till it flows trippingly from your tongue.

Adult day care also tends to be transitional, and the idea works best if your sibling already has somebody living in, usually a spouse, child, or other relative. It's designed to get people who would otherwise be housebound out into the world a bit for interaction with others and perhaps a field trip or two.

Transportation may or may not be available and hours are usually limited to daytime. There is generally some scheduling flexibility and it isn't automatically a 40-hour program. Meals are provided, along with adult supervision and planned activities.

The other function of adult day care, of course, is to give the beleaguered caregiving team some respite. It may be possible to sell the idea more easily to a reluctant invalid if you emphasize that whoever is involved in caregiving absolutely, positively, needs a break.

Don't be afraid to make your sibling feel a little guilty if it will help everybody here.

WHEN LIVING ALONE IS NO LONGER POSSIBLE

At a certain point, it may become clear to everybody that your sibling can't continue in the current living situation. This may be because she's alone and confused, with a tendency to wander or forget medications and meals. Perhaps her house has several flights of narrow, crooked stairs, and she's now in a wheelchair without funds to renovate. Or maybe she had another heart attack.

A new medical event often precipitates the next stage, particularly if it represents a sharp decline of some sort. At this point there are two different paths which may be followed.

One is institutional long term care: assisted living, ideally in a facility where moving to skilled nursing is an easy option in the case of further decline. Sometimes a medical event may eliminate the assisted living stage altogether, sending your sister directly to a skilled nursing facility, or nursing home.

This usually involves moving the patient.

The patient's move may be forestalled if a relative is willing and able to move in as a regular caregiver, but that is also a significant event that will require a lot of adjustments on everybody's part. Or it may be necessary for the patient to move in with a child, sibling, or other friend or relative. (Friends, in these situations, tend not to offer permanent accommodations.)

If a relative is moving in, for heaven's sake take a trial run first, before things get too complicated. And keep in mind that nearly every situation in which moving is involved will involve some downsizing and plenty of stress.

A STRANGER MOVES IN

If that heading has a melodramatic feel, it's no accident.

A surprisingly common fantasy among otherwise reasonable people is the notion that somebody you've never met before will want to move into your sibling's home and serve as caregiver and general factotum in exchange for room and board. This notion has roots in the British institution of the companion, a gentlewoman of limited or reduced means who sees to the needs of a considerably more affluent gentlewoman. (Remember the narrator of *Rebecca*?)

My brother's health crisis occurred against the backdrop of a national financial meltdown. My sister was convinced that we'd have no trouble finding a temporarily down-on-his-luck hedge fund executive or mortgage banker who'd want to move into my brother's house, take him to medical appointments, supervise medications, handle general household maintenance, and finish up a bunch of incomplete renovation projects—all while doing some serious male-bonding over pizza and football.

That plan had innumerable flaws, starting with two basic realities: There was nothing approximating a second bedroom for this person to move into, and we had no obvious way to find, vet, or supervise him, being some 1,800 miles distant.

Also, of course, my brother hated the idea. He didn't even want somebody coming in twice a week, much less invading his personal space.

A more common notion is the idea of finding a college student. Or, if you're really lucky, a nursing student. If you have access to a college community, this one is actually possible, though students are not always the world's most reliable people, or willing to sign on for the long haul.

If you really want to move somebody into your sister's house, the safest solution by far is to bite the bullet and find somebody who is bonded, preferably through a reliable agency. This is bound to cost more than you think it should, but it beats having her wake up one morning to find the companion gone, along with the giant flat screen and Great-Grandma's silver.

MEDICARE AND LONG-TERM CARE

This section will be very brief. Medicare does not cover long-term care. Period.

In some instances, Medicare will pay for limited time in a skilled nursing facility following hospitalization, generally when somebody lives alone and requires a bit of transition. Physical therapy needs may also land somebody in skilled nursing. But there are definite end dates on these services.

Need-based Medicaid may cover long-term care in certain circumstances.

LONG-TERM CARE INSURANCE

Whether you're dealing with a chronic, ongoing situation or a fast breaking crisis, if your sister doesn't already have long-term care insurance, that ship has probably sailed. It may be worth looking into for yourself, but you'll need to find some other way to pay for her.

If she does have coverage, be aware of its terms and understand what is and isn't covered before you lock into costly arrangements. And yes, there will be an ocean of paperwork.

MEMORY IMPAIRMENT

If memory impairment is (or is likely to become) an issue, bump this to the top of your priority list as you look into assisted living facilities. Having your brother familiar with a place before he moves into the Memory Unit may make that transition a lot easier for him. And just knowing that the Memory Unit is there will make the entire process easier for you.

Dementia and memory impairment are providing new challenges for all levels of caregiving, by virtue of sheer numbers. Almost half the people living in nursing homes have some form of dementia, and facilities for the memory-impaired are popping up everywhere as those numbers rise.

You're hoping it will never happen, of course. And maybe it won't, because he's been incredibly lucky so far in a lot of ways. Just the same, it's one bet you may be able to hedge, and if so, that's a great idea.

ASSISTED LIVING

Assisted living is often confused with skilled nursing facilities, AKA nursing homes. The two are anything but identical. To further confuse matters, assisted living has a bunch of other names: residential care, board and care, congregate care, alternative care facilities, group homes, or sheltered housing.

These facilities are licensed by the states in which they exist, and may vary in many ways from one part of the country to another. For that matter, they may vary widely from one side of town to another. Where they are generally the same is in providing a private room or small apartment to residents, offering group activities and exercise, providing meals, and helping with areas where residents require ... assistance.

You generally move your own furniture into an assisted living unit, which is of course perfect for continuity of some sort. Usually there's a little fridge for the Ben and Jerry's. Sometimes you can even bring along your small dog or cat.

Generally a form of needs assessment, again varying from state to state, determines whether somebody requires sufficient help to be eligible for residence. Somebody who has a lot of trouble moving physically but manages her own investment portfolio and sings first soprano at the Presbyterian church may have the same eligibility score as the fellow who can manage a four-mile hike but won't be able to tell you where he went or what he saw.

The needs assessment may also reveal that the prospective resident's problems are too complex or advanced for this setting, and may require skipping directly to a nursing home. That's something to keep in mind, actually. People who fear the idea of being in a nursing home and consequently fight assisted living may find themselves in a nursing home anyway, under circumstances they can't control at all, while somebody else decides what to do with the prized possessions they were unwilling to give up.

When I was interviewing the director of the Southern Illinois assisted living facility where my brother eventually moved, I was dismayed by the thick stack of applications on her desk from people ahead of him in line. There were only two dozen total rooms available, after all, and the folks I'd passed eating lunch in the dining area all looked pretty spry to me. How could we possibly wait that long?

The waiting list was deceptive, the director told me. Each time a room came available, she would call all those applicants, in order. Some of them she'd been calling for years. They'd tell her they weren't quite ready yet, or Christmas was coming and it would be too disruptive right now, or maybe next year after....

And sure enough, when I got the call a month later that a room was coming available and did we want it, it was mid-December. Sleigh bells were ringing, and everybody ahead of us on the list had taken a pass one more time.

I said yes immediately and drove to the post office to get off a check and seal the deal. He moved in a week before Christmas. He wasn't happy about it, to be sure, but he was *there*.

In his own room with his own stuff. Safe.

MAKING CHOICES

Selecting an assisted living facility can be complicated and demoralizing, and it needs to be done in person. Your sister doesn't have to go around to every place in town with you, but she should have the opportunity to visit your top choice or choices and be in on the decision. This is a really difficult transition for most people to make, and the more you can involve her in a positive way, the easier it will be for everyone.

Like other matters of real estate, a lot of the cost of assisted living is a function of location. And none of it is particularly affordable, though the daily cost of my brother's room and board came to less than I paid to spend a night in the unremarkable local hotel.

Try to think the process through before you get too deeply involved, and to match your sibling to the locally-available options.

Your sister may enjoy the activities and camaraderie in a larger facility with a nice dining room and plenty of group opportunities and events. Or she might be a more private person, better suited to a place with fewer residents in a household-type setting, essentially a group home. These places offer intimacy and closer relationships between staff and residents, though that intimacy can be a problem if she doesn't like the other half-dozen residents.

The model for this is the type of group home where developmentally disabled adults often live, perhaps sharing bedrooms or bathrooms, interacting in communal areas, eating together, and supervised by a live-in manager. These places aren't always perfect, heaven knows, but the biggest complaint I hear on the SibNet list is that there aren't enough of them.

The same model has also been used very successfully for patients living with HIV/AIDS. At one point when my brother's condition was in breakneck decline and his living options still totally unsettled, I happened to attend the 20th Anniversary Party for Fraternity House, a San Diego group home which had initially offered dignity and hospice to men with AIDS who had nowhere else to go.

After two decades, all that had changed dramatically. Now people were recovering sufficiently to go back out into the world, a year had just passed without a single resident's death, and one of the guys in the band playing in the living room was a former resident.

At that moment, I recognized what a perfect solution such a place could be for folks of my generation with various physical problems. Everybody gets their own rooms, nobody has to cook who doesn't want to, and there's somebody on-site in the background to handle medical matters.

My own circle of college friends has long envisioned us hanging out on the porch of our own group home, talking quietly into the night.

Or maybe not so quietly; our hearing isn't quite what it used to be.

A POSITIVE SPIN FROM
AN UNEXPECTED QUARTER

As I began this chapter, one of my writer friends posted on Facebook about taking an aunt to tour an assisted living facility and discovering it to be "writer heaven." Others chimed in immediately about the writer-friendly perks: private room, full food and dining room service, library, cleaning service, shuttle bus to take you where you need to go, exercise equipment, and in some places the option to keep a small pet.

In short, a place where all you need to do is enjoy your own activities, either privately or with your buddies.

So try focusing on that element if you possibly can.

NURSING HOMES

Nursing homes or skilled nursing facilities provide services to patients whose needs are far greater than residents of assisted living facilities. This care is not cheap. The median price for a year in a private room of a nursing home is now $84,000. And that's assuming you can locate a place you consider satisfactory, in the appropriate geographic area.

There are other issues.

Nursing homes conjure images of nasty smells and patients bent over all day in wheelchairs, drooling. Of blaring communal TV. Of thieving night staff and dementia-driven residents requiring restraints. Of inadequate safety precautions such as sprinkler systems. Of bedsores and teeth unbrushed for months.

What's unfortunate is that there is truth in all of this. These things do all happen, here and there. You *do* need to be particularly careful in selecting a nursing home, if indeed selection is possible. Sometimes there aren't a lot of choices, particularly if you live in a sparsely populated area or are dependent on Medicaid for payment.

So you need to focus on the best ways to insure your sibling's safety and well-being.

Getting chummy with the staff is always useful, and

bringing (or sending) candy or flowers for the front office is a capital idea. Spot check at odd times. One of the biggest issues just now in the nursing home world is nanny cams, which relatives of some patients are installing to be more comfortable about the care their loved ones receive. Privacy issues intrude here if your sister has a roommate whose family objects to that type of surveillance.

Things are slightly more complicated if you've waited (or if your brother has refused to move) until dementia was established. It's already a tough call to place a loved one in a nursing home, and with dementia there tends to be more guilt and less societal understanding, at least in part because he may look just fine and others don't see the behaviors that have you worried sick.

Another concern is that you can't depend on somebody with dementia to report (or even notice) inappropriate or negligent behavior.

Meanwhile, you may find people thinking (or even worse, saying): *What kind of shiftless bum can't take care of this dear sweet guy at home?* And while it's really none of their business, you feel compelled to try to explain. And so on.

Nobody wants to be in a nursing home. Nobody plans to be in a nursing home.

Sometimes there just isn't a choice.

ADDITIONAL INFORMATION

General Information

AARP Livable Communities Resources
www.aarp.org/livable-communities/

The Cohousing Association of the United States
www.cohousing.org/

Cohousing California
www.calcoho.org/

The Cohousing Company
www.cohousingco.com/

Eldercare Locator
www.eldercare.gov
800.677.1116

LeadingAge: Center for Housing Plus Services
www.leadingage.org/Center_for_Housing_Plus_Services.aspx

National Center for Assisted Living
www.ahcancal.org/ncal/Pages/index.aspx

Senior Resource Housing Choices for Seniors
www.seniorresource.com/house.htm

Long-Term Care

Guide to Long-Term Care for Veterans
www.va.gov/GERIATRICS/Guide/LongTermCare/index.asp

Homecare Online: How to Choose a Home Care Provider
www.nahc.org/consumer-information/right-home-care-provider/

Long-Term Care
www.longtermcare.com

National Clearinghouse for Long-Term Care Information
www.longtermcare.gov

Visiting Nurse Associations of America
vnaa.org/
888.866.8773

• • • • •

Harley Gordon
In Sickness & in Health: How to Discuss and Create a Plan for Long-Term Care and the Consequences to Your Family and Finances if You Don't
Financial Strategies Press, 2007

Dan Keppel
Long-Term Care Insurance: Is It Right for You? Are There Better Alternatives?
Amazon Kindle, 2012

Joseph L. Matthews
Long-Term Care: How to Plan & Pay for It, 9th Edition
Nolo, 2012

Joseph L. Matthews
Long-Term Care Insurance: Do You Need It?
Nolo eBook only

Phyllis Shelton
Long-Term Care: Your Financial Planning Guide, 9th Edition
LTCi Publishing, 2008

Peter S. Silin
Nursing Homes and Assisted Living: The Family's Guide to Making Decisions and Getting Good Care, 2nd Edition
Johns Hopkins Press, 2009

Robyn Stone
Long-Term Care for the Elderly
Urban Institute, 2011

Jeff Tomlin
Will I Need Long-Term Care? LTC Planning Guide and Workbook
CreateSpace, 2013

ACCESSIBILITY, MODIFICATIONS, AND ASSISTIVE TECHNOLOGY

Many serious medical conditions will require modifications in lifestyle and living quarters.

Whether these are short-term or long-term, they often present challenges that you simply never thought about before. Everybody has encountered people using wheelchairs, for instance, but until somebody close to you actually has to use one you don't consider issues such as turning radius, door width, and level of incline.

These are highly individualized situations, so what we'll deal with here are general problems, simple solutions, and how to find further information. The things to keep in mind as you consider changes are safety, independence, and flexibility.

Some of the larger and costlier items are available through or can be partially funded by Medicare and/or other governmental or disease-related agencies. Be sure to check on this before plunking down a mountain of cash for something you never heard of before last Friday.

The potential for government financing may lead to fairly aggressive sales levels, as those who watch late-night TV can attest. Express even a slight interest in a particular type of aid and you are likely to find ads for it on your Facebook page and a blizzard of emails from companies offering Just What You Need. At one point I filled in an online request to have printed information about walk-in bathtubs mailed to me and within five minutes my phone was ringing with a sales rep eager to help. Tell those people to put you on their Do Not Call list if you don't want to be bothered by them; they are required by law to obey and penalties can be harsh.

Some modifications are absurdly expensive and others ridiculously cheap. For the most part there is an option for every budget and when that isn't the case, various agencies and community organizations may be able to help.

LONG TERM OR SHORT TERM?

Many of the decisions you make in these areas will be based on whether your sibling's problem is likely to be short-term but intense; long-term and possibly chronic; or long-term and progressive.

Be careful here. Everybody's initial inclination may be that this is a short-term, easy-fix kind of situation and that she will be running marathons in a few months (assuming that she ran them in the first place). Positive attitude is always important, but don't let it get in the way of realism.

On the other hand, if you know that major long-term modifications are going to be necessary, try not to panic and make hasty decisions before you have sufficient information and perspective. Think things through and discuss the problems and challenges with others on the team.

Remember to enlist input from any physical or occupational therapists your sister is working with. You are dealing with one person but these people work with many people sharing similar problems. They can be invaluable resources for tips on local assistance and government and/or private agencies that work with these problems. They are also excellent sources for feedback on what *doesn't* work.

Be sure to also check early on with your local Council on Independent Living (CIL) or Statewide Independent Living Council (SILC), which will have both general suggestions and resources applicable to where you are. Links to these are at: www.ilru.org/.

GENERAL ACCESSIBILITY

The gold standard in this area is a slim volume by Shelley Peterman Schwarz called *Home Accessibility: 300 Tips for Making Life Easier,* supplemented by her companion website www.makinglifeeasier.com. Schwarz came to this topic the hard way, with a diagnosis of MS at the age of 32, and has also written volumes dealing with specific problems of Multiple Sclerosis, Parkinson's, and arthritis. Her website updates all this material, offers a newsletter, and is all but guaranteed to offer ideas that might never have occurred to you.

GETTING AROUND THE HOUSE

First things first.

Is getting in and out of the house a problem all by itself? Maybe that flight of outside stairs didn't seem like much when everybody was sprinting up and down it twenty years ago. For somebody with crutches, a walker, a cane, or a wheelchair, it may as well be Mount Everest, and that's before it even starts to snow. Inside stairs can be equally problematic to somebody with balance or walking issues.

If somebody has a short-term physical problem and there's space available elsewhere that isn't so stairs-challenged (like in another family member's home), consider a brief move. You may also want to move a bedroom down to the ground floor on either a temporary or permanent basis. One reason why people are sometimes sent from hospitals to rehab facilities instead of directly home is that they simply can't get into or around that home just now.

Be sure to install railings and grab bars anyplace that's iffy. This includes every stairway going anywhere (basements and attics are easy to overlook and can be treacherous) and if there are likely to be long-term climbing issues, you probably should have railings on both sides of all major staircases. These can be so unobtrusive that they aren't even noticeable.

Doorways in many buildings aren't wide enough to easily accommodate wheelchairs and even getting a walker through a narrow doorway can be an adventure. Doors may open the wrong way for easy mobility or have some kind of obstruction on one side. In a pinch, consider taking a difficult door off its hinges for a while.

You may want to think about temporarily repurposing space. A computer can be moved out of the upstairs home office into a more convenient spot, for instance, even if you aren't moving the bedroom downstairs.

Keep pathways clear! It's tough enough when you can't get around easily, without worrying about tripping on … well, anything and everything. If there are throw rugs, pack them up for the duration or get rid of them. Little tables holding little knick-knacks are a recipe for disaster. Move them out, or at least well out of the way.

For somebody with vision problems, stair risers on the back of each step may be difficult to distinguish from the treads where you set your feet. Risers can be painted a different color from the treads, and if that doesn't seem workable, you can use a temporary fix of blue painter's tape along the stair edge. Same thing for the junction where wall meets floor, or where a freestanding wall turns a corner.

Somebody who's using a walker or wheelchair can't easily run back to the kitchen or bedroom for a forgotten item. Trick out that wheeled vehicle the same way you did your bike, with a basket to hold frequently used items. Bags are designed to slip over arms of wheelchairs to hold stuff and the seating area on walkers with that option usually conceals storage space that can be used for an extra pair of glasses, reading material, a cell phone or a tablet, snacks, and just about anything else that would normally require getting up and fetching.

And don't forget a cup holder.

GETTING IN AND OUT OF ROOMS

Doorknobs can be cantankerous—unwilling to turn for somebody with arthritis or too slippery or hard to reach for somebody using a walker or wheelchair. Outside doorknobs or locks that involve keys can also be absurdly challenging.

Home Accessibility identifies all kinds of ways to simplify door problems, including an E-Z Pull Door Closer which is inexpensive and easily installed on any door. Rubber door knob grippers are a big help for almost anybody who has difficulty gripping and turning a knob. If you don't have to worry about having an interior door securely latched, you might want to slap some tape across the tongue like the Watergate burglars. Then you can use hanging pulls on both sides.

RAMPS

Ramps may seem like an easy answer for somebody who can't manage stairs, but be sure they are put in by somebody who knows the local building code and also understands how to do it correctly. If your brother-in-law nails a 4x8 piece of plywood at a 45-degree angle over the front steps, you're looking at a runaway wheelchair, a spectacular header, and a trip to the emergency room with lights flashing.

Ramps may not be optional, particularly if there is a progressive or permanent physical impediment. In that case, you'll want to go to a fair amount of trouble so that any new ramp is consistent with the rest of the building, relatively unobtrusive, wide enough, railed on both sides, and at a gentle enough grade that nobody will fly off the side on the way down or require a Scout troop working in unison to push the chair to the top.

Textured paint or paint with sand mixed into it will help create a rougher surface to prevent slips and falls. And make sure the whole business is adequately lit.

REACHING THINGS

The two obvious ways to deal with accessing hard-to-reach objects are to move them to a more manageable location (always preferable) or use a reacher. These simple mechanical devices extend an arm for a couple more feet with a claw that grasps objects on the business end. I have several, keep them in different rooms, and use them frequently to get things down from high shelves or awkward locations.

You may find some initial resistance to this, but reachers grow on you pretty quickly. You may need to try a couple of different styles to find the one that works best for you. A reacher can usually be attached fairly easily to a walker or wheelchair as well.

I have often wished I had a reacher with me in the grocery store, and loved learning that the popular series character Jack Reacher got his name because the author, Lee Child, is extremely tall and was frequently asked to get down high items in public places. Before he became a mega-bestselling author, his wife suggested that if the book business didn't work out, he could hire himself out as a reacher.

GENERAL TECHNOLOGY

Voice activation is extremely useful for people with temporary or progressive difficulty in small motor skills. You can get your tablet, television, alarm clock, and just about anything else to turn itself on or off with the right technical aids. As for telephones, Siri and her android cousins will cheerfully take care of all kinds of matters for you on a smartphone, and all you have to do is issue simple instructions.

Remote control devices are ubiquitous, and if your brother is having difficulty manipulating the platoon lined up by his television, think big and simple. You can get a universal remote with numbers that you can read from the next room and that can be easily punched by somebody who's having difficulty with finger control. People have strong emotional connections to the way they use their remotes, so there are likely to be transition issues here, but once you get the new one set up properly, everybody should be happier.

In a related vein, if handling a cell phone with its tiny screen and tinier keypad has become more difficult, consider a Jitterbug. My brother had one when his small motor skills went missing and it worked quite well for him.

The Jitterbug was developed for seniors and it's easy to use. It's larger than most flip phones, has a keypad with great big numbers, and is designed to be very intuitive. You answer questions "Yes" or "No" and it takes care of the rest. Voice mail, texting, and assisted dialing are available.

In fact, there's now a Jitterbug smartphone, which seems almost oxymoronic. The Jitterbug Touch3 has a large flat screen, limited and easily accessed options, and will work nicely for somebody who either can't manage his own smartphone any more or who wants to have access to additional features. Some of those include health and medical apps, as well as a daily check-in call service. Both the flip and touch-screen models have built-in cameras.

At the opposite end, the Splash model is strictly a cry for assistance, a waterproof fall detector with a single-button to be pushed for help.

Since Great Call's Jitterbug system piggybacks on other carriers for its reception, it may even have better coverage than what you're accustomed to right now.

BATHROOMS

Bathrooms are slippery places under the best of circumstances, and major safety concerns the rest of the time. The combination of water and hard flooring in a confined space (plus sharp edges, glass accoutrements, and soap) contributes to a disproportionately high rate of household falls and accidents. Given the tightness-of-space issue, bathrooms are excellent candidates for temporary door removal, particularly in master suites.

The good news is that a lot of bathroom safety issues can be mitigated fairly easily. A rustproof, rubber-footed chair in the tub or shower and an extended shower handle are a cheap and easy start. Generous use of stick-on safety tape or tub designs will ease the risk of general slippage in tub, shower, and even on the floor. Grab bars are relatively easy to install and probably ought to be in any tub or shower anyway. Remember to thoroughly rinse soap residue off all surfaces.

Keep items used in the shower in a basket with a handle (the same kind used by kids living in dorms) to simplify matters. Store other frequently-used bathroom items in a single, easily accessible drawer to eliminate the need to bend, reach, or rummage around. Nightlights are essential both in the bathroom and the areas leading to it, and if concern about balance or falls is high, leaving some kind of small light on all night may be a good idea. A motion sensor light can be just the ticket here.

If you are looking at long-term modifications, consider a walk-in bathtub. These are quite expensive and you can't just slap one in place, but if somebody has new mobility issues that aren't likely to improve a lot, it may allow him to continue enjoying a good soak without risking a concussion getting in and out of the tub.

A raised toilet seat with or without side rails is an easily-installed fix and makes all kinds of things simpler, as do various toilet hygiene accessories such as wipe assisters and spritzers. Since the Greatest Generation lived so long, there's now a world of continence materials available both at the supermarket and more specialized supply companies.

And make sure all concerned know that flushing commercial wipes is a dandy way to clog pipes. You have enough going on without emergency calls to the plumber.

BEDROOMS

The new realities of your sister's health may dictate that she will be spending a lot more time in the bedroom than she's been accustomed to. If this is a short-term issue, simple modifications may do the trick, and if it's longer-lasting you may want to rent or buy a hospital bed.

Hospital beds aren't pretty, and they also represent a psychological insertion of unwelcome technology into the ultimate refuge and sanctuary of the bedroom. Some people get around this issue by buying a mattress system with head and foot that raise and lower, a pricey but more attractive solution. You can also get sturdy blow-up wedges that insert between a (flexible) mattress and box spring or you may choose to rely on wedge-shaped pillows.

Tables that slide under the bed and have a tray on top are useful for somebody who's going to be there a while and needs a handy spot to set things. These can roll away easily when they're not needed and don't have to look like their familiar metal and Formica cousins from the hospital.

If the bed is too low, risers are a fast and easy solution. These look like heavy-duty ice cream or cottage cheese containers and go under the four corners of the bed for a fast six-inch hoist. When I got mine some years ago, they were a novelty item available only in a few catalogues, but they're now commonly found in bedding departments all over the place.

Conversely, if the bed is too high and your sister isn't in shape to be make a flying leap up into it, you might consider steps. However, if the steps seem more dangerous than making that leap, perhaps it's time to switch out a charming but rickety antique four-poster for something more functional. If the bed has been in the family forever, maybe it can move to a guest bedroom or go to a favorite niece. Or you can take it apart and store it in the basement or attic.

Be sure there's a decent, easily-turned-on reading lamp beside the bed and a good remote if the bedroom has a television. If it doesn't have TV, consider running a new line to offer that to the patient. Lighting becomes more critical if somebody's going to be in bed for a while, so check carefully in the section below for other options and issues.

Since it's unlikely that your sister is fully utilizing her wardrobe at the moment, place the items she *is* wearing regularly together in an easily accessed drawer or comfortably-reached section of the closet. Frequently-worn shoes or slippers can go right there on the floor by the bed.

KITCHENS

Your sibling may welcome this excuse to get out of the kitchen, but it's a tough room to avoid if you want to eat. How much or how little you need to adapt here depends on how the kitchen was used in the first place.

If your brother has been in the habit of nuking a frozen dinner each night whether he's hungry or not, make sure he can reach the stash in the freezer (reacher tools are perfect for this) and can easily access the microwave. Position a trash can at a convenient spot and you're done.

If your sister enjoys cooking and likes to work in the

kitchen, then have her figure out which pots, bowls, utensils and dishes she uses most often and clear out a cabinet to put them all in one easily-accessed location. Ditto commonly used ingredients, condiments, and seasonings. She might not want the turmeric or walnut oil every night, but she's likely to have a favorite knife, salt shaker, and a few other things she uses constantly.

If standing for long periods (or at all) is a new problem for a dedicated cook, try a padded floor mat, find a stool that's a comfortable height for counter work, or relocate the whole process to the kitchen table where the cook can sit in comfort. If you're moving the operation, stash those frequently-used items nearby in a cupboard or on a rolling cart.

If handling kitchen tools is difficult, look into the OXO soft-handled utensils which were designed for people with arthritis and other problems gripping.

LIGHTS

All kinds of timers can be used to keep a living space appropriately lit without anybody having to literally lift a finger. In main parts of the home, you can set timers to go on half an hour before sunset and to go off half an hour after your sister usually goes to bed and you're done. If it's winter and she's an early riser, new timers will happily allow you to set multiple on/off times.

Bedside and/or reading lights can be connected to mechanisms that are remote controlled, or touch-the-lamp-base controlled, or even voice-controlled. Remember those irritating commercials for the Clapper? "Clap—ON!! Clap—OFF!!" Couldn't be simpler.

Motion sensors around the exterior of the house will turn on lighting when they're disturbed, such as when somebody approaches the front door. Indoors, motion sensors can be particularly useful for middle-of-the-night bathroom expeditions. And it goes without saying (though I'm going to say it anyway) that you want the path to the bathroom well lit.

Nightlights in lesser-used areas of the house use almost

no power, particularly if you get the sensor kind that turn themselves on only when it's dark. These may seem like overkill but if somebody needs to venture into a part of the house that's off the customary path, it's nice to be able to see where you're going. Keep a light on in the kitchen at night if the person may need crackers or water to alleviate upset stomachs from meds.

Stairways should be clearly lit on both ends as well as in the middle. And if you're worried about somebody taking an inadvertent tumble down the stairs, a gate across the top is a dandy idea. Since folks are using these to keep pets as well as small children out of certain areas these days, there are very attractive options that don't look like a playpen.

Consider outdoor solar lighting that doesn't have to be hooked up to anything. Solar has gotten both better and cheaper in recent years. You might light a porch with larger solar lamps, or line a pathway with a bunch of the small ones. In Southern states, this can be a year-round system, though up north heavy snow and scant sunlight may render them useless for part of the year. Even there, however, they'll be handy on summer paths.

And for the ultimate in gracious living under duress, some battery-operated candles will turn themselves on and off at the same time every day.

It's easy to get carried away with lighting, but it's a lot better than having to deal with the aftermath of a bad fall resulting from a poorly lit stairway or bathroom.

ASSISTIVE TECHNOLOGY, WHATEVER THAT IS

Suzanne Robitaille's *The Illustrated Guide to Assistive Technology and Devices* is chock full of information about the technical types of equipment you may need to make life more manageable. Unfortunately, it's several years old in a field with hourly updates and not readily available except in digital form, though that seems appropriate enough.

Robitaille also came to her expertise the hard way, having grown up profoundly deaf before receiving a cochlear implant at the age of twenty-seven. She maintains a regularly updated website, Abled Body: abledbody.com/

Assistive Technology is defined differently (but with great authority) on all kinds of lists put together by all kinds of different people, and also has a silly overblown government definition written in legalese. Basically it's anything technical or mechanical that makes life easier for somebody who's got any kind of physical, mental, or emotional problem.

AIR QUALITY

In general, breathing problems build up over a period of time. However, if somebody has been in poor health (and also perhaps in denial about that poor health) and chronic lung problems are involved, you might be looking at several related problems.

One of these may be the condition of the patient's natural environment.

If that's the case, getting herds of dust buffaloes out of your sibling's home and creating an easier-to-care-for environment becomes urgent. Bring in family reinforcements and make it a day's project with pizza and peppy music if there are enough bodies to be useful. (Two can be enough if they're the right two. Or if the alternative is doing it yourself.) This might also be a good time to call on non-relatives or distant kinfolk who've asked what they can do to help.

If all else fails, hire a maid service.

Once again, the throw rugs need to go, along with dust-catchers in general. The object is to remove the dust, not rearrange it. Hard floors are better than carpet. Carpet that needs to stay must be frequently vacuumed and ought to be steam-cleaned at the outset. None of this is rocket science.

In my childhood, air cleanliness wasn't discussed and cigarettes smoldered in ashtrays everywhere. It's a whole new world, with a breathtaking selection of air cleaning machinery and concepts. Check with your brother's pulmonary specialist for recommendations, and read up on ratings and reviews for how well they actually work.

Change filters regularly.

Anything that pushes air around needs to be regularly cleaned, and anything with a filter needs to have that filter cleaned or changed at frequent intervals.

That's air cleaners, furnaces, air conditioners, fans, and vents. These systems work by pulling air in on one side and pushing it out on another. The filter's job is to trap the crud in that air. As crud builds up in the filter, the equipment works less efficiently and you increase the likelihood that some of the smaller crud particles will get pushed through and go right back into circulation.

You might consider having somebody clean the ducts in a forced-air heating or cooling system. When people slide through them in movie thrillers, they're always slick and shiny and clean, but in real life matters tend to be grungier. I've had my ducts cleaned by a chimney sweep, just like Mary Poppins.

House plants can also help improve air quality, removing formaldehyde and other toxins from the atmosphere while adding oxygen. There's even an official list of NASA-approved houseplants for the Space Shuttle. Many of the best performers here are readily available, cheap, and hardy, including philodendrons, English ivy, dracaenas, pothos, and rubber plant. Those who claim black thumbs might at least consider snake plant (also known as Mother-in-law's Tongue and cast iron plant), because it is extremely hardy and in the habit of producing oxygen at night when other plants are resting. This makes it a particularly good choice for bedrooms.

Houseplants will only be useful, however, if somebody is going to pay some kind of regular attention. Dead sticks just collect more dust.

VISION AIDS AND SUPPLEMENTS

The American Foundation for the Blind has a world of information about how to deal with vision problems, and has also developed plenty of technology products itself, from insulin pens to voting machines. Their extremely comprehensive website includes sections on Adapting Your

Home. Start with the major menu choice "Living with Vision Loss" on the website and go from there. www.afb.org/ In addition, VisionAware features extensive ideas and suggestions in their section on Everyday Living. www.visionaware.org

People with gradually developing vision problems can call upon all manner of magnification devices, most far more task-specific than the familiar Sherlock Holmes magnifying glass. This is how most folks with deteriorating vision ease into their new reality, and it works as well now as it did when Great-Grandma was threading her needle.

In an information age, losing the ability to read can be devastating to somebody who has been accustomed to relying on the printed word. Macular degeneration, another one of those afflictions people weren't widely aware of last century, is a serious contributor to this problem. Luckily, technology has stepped into this breach and opened all kinds of new options.

Not long ago, people who were blind or had very low vision were limited to the world of Braille books, reel-to-reel tape recordings, and Talking Books provided with special recorders by the American Foundation for the Blind.

Braille books are cumbersome volumes that are "read" by touching fingers to combinations of raised dots representing letters. These dots are literally punched into the pages, which are the color and weight of manila file folders. It takes a lot of space to make a word that can be read by fingertips and a whole lot more for sentences, paragraphs and chapters. Braille books are extremely bulky.

I took piano lessons as a child from a blind woman whose numerous blind students worked exclusively with Braille music, bulkier than telephone books. These students were significantly more talented than I, however, so perhaps their not being able to simultaneously read and play music wasn't the obstacle it would have been for some of us.

Electronic media have made a wide range of books available to the visually challenged, as well as to the rest of us. Back in the 1960s when my mother was reading specific books into a reel-to-reel tape recorder by request for clients of Illinois Tape Recording for the Blind, this was not an option. I read a book for them one college summer, a history of the slave trade that I thought would be interesting. It was, but it was also nearly 500 pages long, and it takes a very long time to read 500 pages out loud.

Then audiocassettes were born, and books on tape followed closely behind, both abridged and unabridged. Today audio books are available as CDs and MP3s and you can download them from library websites and listen to them on your phone. You can also, of course, purchase all these types of audio books, and listen to them on a wide array of devices no matter what the state of your vision might be.

Large print books are available for a narrow range of titles deemed to be of interest to those with visual impairment or advancing years, two categories that tend to move in tandem. These books are available for purchase and in libraries, and are usually quite expensive.

The advent of e-readers has also made print reading much easier for those with severe vision problems. You can easily adjust the size of the font of a book on most e-readers to be as big as it needs to be—even if that leaves four words on a page.

People with vision issues in Southern California should also check out the Braille Institute. Free Low Vision Consultations are available to those with referrals from a health care professional. These are conducted one-on-one by appointment at five Southern California locations. www.brailleinstitute.org/

The Lighthouse Guild offers an incredible array of products designed to simplify life for those with vision impairment. www.lighthouseguild.org/programs-services/store

HEARING ASSISTANCE

Reluctance to admit hearing issues is nothing new. Just about everybody had a great uncle who insisted there was nothing wrong with his hearing even when folks had to shout like cartoon characters to get his attention.

The obvious solution to many hearing problems is

hearing aids, which are no longer big clunky things that clap on to the back of an ear. Now they're often tiny enough to fit inside the ear itself, and so many people are attached to ear buds and iPods and Bluetooth devices for cell phones that nobody is likely to even notice something in somebody else's ear.

Assistive Technology and Devices offers over forty pages of material related to hearing problems, starting with materials designed for those not yet ready to use hearing aids. All kinds of amplification devices are available, including assistive living systems (ALSs) used for communication between the person with the hearing problem and somebody else. Check AbleData.com for additional current possibilities.

Signaling devices that flash bright lights when the bell is rung can be connected to doorbells. An aunt who emerged deaf from a bout with sepsis had one of these, and the first time I saw it in action it reminded me of a flashing fire truck. Other devices rely on vibration, including alarm clocks that shake the bed.

Closed-captioning for television and movies has been around a long time, and the primary issue is generally accuracy. Simultaneous translations to text (as with news programming) are sometimes awkward, summarize to fit the info, tend to run a bit behind the visuals, and occasionally make blunders that are hilarious if you aren't relying on them for solid information.

DVDs come automatically with closed-caption options, but HD-DVD and Blu-ray technology has lagged behind, and not all media with closed-captioning will play on all equipment. Be sure to check on compatibility if making new purchases.

Text telephones (TTY) are also old news, upstaged by recent developments in both telephone and computer technologies. Email and instant messaging (IM) are just as easy as a TTY machine and can be accessed almost anywhere. So can run-of-the-mill texting, the sleek contemporary grandchild of the old TTY machinery.

COMPUTERS

The good news about computer technology is that it advances on a daily basis. That's also the bad news, since the development that seems too good to be true in January may be obsolete by March.

If your sister is not at ease with computers or prides herself on being a technological luddite, this is probably not the time to insist that she embrace 21st Century technology. But if she's been comfortably using a computer, adding bells and whistles to deal with specific new problems may be quite simple. She already knows what she wants to do on her computer, after all, so you can work backward from her new physical problems.

Working backward is relatively easy. Determine what you want to do and then look for the best way to do it. If you know somebody who is already operating a particular system or using a type of program successfully, you're ahead of the game. If vision is an issue, a large monitor can be added to any system (including a laptop) and keyboard adjustments will increase fonts to whatever size you need. Keyboards designed for particular problems (visual or manual) are available and AbleData.com has dozens of listings for both hardware and software solutions. They even list materials that are no longer available for reference purposes.

Touchscreen technology that is currently used in tablets and smartphones can be very helpful, particularly if your sister is already familiar with it. Modifications for tablets include keyboards and virtual keyboards that are projected onto a large flat space to avoid fumbling with too-small keys.

Voice activated systems have been around for a while and may solve problems for somebody with newly-developed dexterity problems, either in the short or long run. Also in the sound department, some websites are set up to read content aloud to you.

If your sister has been limping along with Windows 95 and a forty-pound monochrome monitor, perhaps this *is* the time to upgrade. Just make sure that she's on board with the decision since computer surprises for the reluctant tend not to have happy endings. And be prepared to work with her as she gets used to her new world, whether this means enlisting a knowledgeable and patient grandchild, enrolling her in a class at the senior center, or hiring a tutor.

ORGANIZING FOR MEMORY IMPAIRMENT

Organizing to simplify matters for somebody with memory impairment is covered in the chapter on "Memory Impairment." The guiding premises are:
- Keep it simple.
- Keep it familiar. Don't set up fancy new systems where everything is in a different place.
- Use labeling wherever possible, either with printed labels or pictures, depending on what you are identifying.

SERVICE DOGS

My blind piano teacher's guide dog Raven was a large and gentle black lab with as placid a disposition as his mistress. Guide dogs were few and far between back then, mostly German Shepherds. In fact, it has only just occurred to me that none of her numerous blind students had guide dogs of their own, which I hope was because they were still technically children.

The novelty has definitely worn off for service animals, which now seem ubiquitous and perform a wide range of assistive services. Service animals tend a wide range of owners with autism, vision or hearing problems, seizures, general mobility issues, and PTSD. For those who need their help, they can help open and reopen entire worlds.

The ADA (Americans with Disabilities Act) says a service animal is "any animal that is individually trained to do work or person tasks for the benefit of a person with a disability." This training is extensive and is provided by the organization which supplies the animal, generally at no charge to the user. That animal is almost always a dog, for fairly obvious reasons related to trainability. Cats wash out in boot camp.

Indeed, the universality of service animals has become something of a problem itself, since there is no official certification beyond paperwork from the training facility. Anybody can go online and buy a vest and tags for Fluffy-the-badly-trained-pet, and then claim the right to take her everywhere. Then when Fluffy pees on the restaurant carpet and jumps on unsuspecting waiters, it gives a bad name to legitimate service animals.

So how can you tell if a service animal is legit? Legally, a business can ask only two questions: Is this a service dog? What is it trained to do for you? Anybody with a genuine service animal will be happy to respond.

A real service animal will probably wear a harness rather than a simple lead, and may or may not have some kind of identifying vest. More to the point, it will not be jumping around, or sniffing your crotch, or licking children, or barking, or lifting a leg in the wrong place. These dogs are trained. Really trained, as in not every animal makes it through the course and there are no awards for Best Self-Esteem in a Golden Retriever Who Means Well.

You should barely be aware of the presence of a service animal, since its entire focus is on assisting the owner.

It's bad karma to try to pass off a pet as a service animal, whether it's your purse dog who offers emotional comfort or your St. Bernard who carries the brandy flask.

DISASTER PLAN

We live in a world where natural disasters sometimes seem to be occurring everywhere simultaneously. Everybody should have at least a general plan for what to do in the case of disaster or emergency.

Your homegrown natural disasters may be hurricanes or tornadoes or earthquakes or blizzards or floods or wildfires, depending on where you live. Nor are these limited to obvious areas any more. Washington, D.C., had an earthquake not long ago, while New Jersey was battered by a hurricane that flooded the New York City subway system.

If your sibling is living alone, it's particularly important to have some kind of plan in place, even if you don't have one set up for yourself. This should include information on who to contact both for immediate assistance and to report being all right. A helpful neighbor might be enlisted to check on your sister when the evacuation order comes, and to be sure that she is taking her medication as well as the daguerreotypes of your forebears and Aunt Elspeth's diamond broach.

It's entirely possible that she had such a plan in place before her medical adventures began, but that may no longer be useful if she's now dependent on a walker and can't remember where the candles are kept. In that case, update the original plan and be sure that anybody likely to be involved in case of emergency knows what it is.

WHERE DO YOU FIND ALL THIS STUFF?

The easiest way to get started here is with a database maintained for the National Institute on Disability and Rehabilitation Research: AbleData.com. Nothing is for sale here but everything is listed, and I do mean everything. Over 200 different products are listed and fully explained under "Caster Shower Chair." Nearly five-dozen drink holders. And if you want to get really specific, how about a Powered Oven Lifter?

Once you know what you want, you can Google the specific product and find out where the best place and price are for you. Don't forget to check Craigslist.org for your community as well. People are often eager to get rid of these things when they no longer need them.

There are also loads of catalogues and websites that specialize in items for people with medical or physical problems and disabilities. They're not all stodgy companies with pictures of nonagenarians, either. I got a catalog of helpful products recently that included a section of remarkably explicit sexual aids.

And as we all know, once you place a single order from any catalogue, your mailbox will be flooded with similar items. If you prefer to eliminate this, you can opt out of any or all catalogues (and other junk mail) at www.catalogchoice.org/.

HOW TO PAY FOR IT ALL

The cost of items discussed in this chapter range from pennies to tens of thousands of dollars. For items deemed medically essential by your sibling's medical team, Medicare and private health insurance will often kick in full or partial payment.

But Medicare isn't going to put in a wheelchair ramp or buy the kickass wheelchair that could compete at the Indy 500, much less the hand-control-operated van into which that chair will be loaded. If your family is short on trillionaires, don't despair.

Look around at your sibling's extended support system, if there is one. Churches and service organizations such as Kiwanis and Rotary are often willing to assist financially, and the service clubs generally don't care if you aren't a member. They may also have able-bodied souls or youth groups willing to help with chores like putting up the storm windows and taking down the awnings.

It doesn't need to be a formal organization, either. Is there a group of old boys who meet every morning at the Dairy Queen and are Vietnam vets like your brother? Try to think creatively and don't be afraid to ask for help. The worst that can happen is somebody will say no, after all, and at least you then have the satisfaction of knowing they probably feel guilty about it.

Churches sometimes maintain a storage area for donated medical items that members no longer need, and while you seek funding for the Parnelli Jones motor chair, there may be a perfectly functional push wheelchair that will serve in the interim. When I helped clear out such a storage area at our church, we found several walkers, two wheelchairs, various commodes, and a cord of crutches.

Look on Craigslist for high ticket items. If somebody bought a hospital bed and no longer needs it, you may be able to get an excellent deal. My sister managed to get two separate computers donated for our brother through ads on Craigslist, and while neither was perfect, the price was certainly right.

ADDITIONAL INFORMATION

General Modifications and Assistive Devices

AbleData: Assistive Technology Products, News, and Resources (Database of specific products and where to find them)
www.abledata.com/

Abled Body (Suzanne Robitaille's website)
www.abledbody.com

Accessible Technology Coalition
www.atcoalition.org/

Center for Accessible Technology
www.cforat.org/

Christopher and Dana Reeve Foundation (Paralysis Resource Center→Assistive Technology)
www.christopherreeve.org/
800.225.0292

Home Modifications
www.homemods.org/

Jitterbug Phones
www.greatcall.com

Making Life Easier: Solutions for Coping with Aging, Chronic Illness or Disability (Shelley Peterman Schwarz's website)
www.makinglifeeasier.com

National Assistive Technology Technical Assistance Partnership (NATTAP)
State-Specific Programs for Assistance Technology Needs
www.resnaprojects.org/nattap/at/stateprograms.html

National Council on Independent Living (links to state and local ICLs)
www.ilru.org/

•••••

Gary Karp
Life on Wheels: The A to Z Guide to Living Fully with Mobility Issues
Demos Health, 2008

Jeffrey C. May and Connie L. May
The Mold Survival Guide: For Your Home and For Your Health
Johns Hopkins University Press, 2004

Suzanne Robitaille
The Illustrated Guide to Assistive Technology & Devices: Tools and Gadgets for Living Independently
Demos Health, 2009

Shelley Peterman Schwarz
Arthritis: 300 Tips for Making Life Easier
Demos Health, 2008

Shelley Peterman Schwarz
Home Accessibility: 300 Tips for Making Life Easier
Demos Health, 2011

Shelley Peterman Schwarz
Multiple Sclerosis: 300 Tips for Making Life Easier
Demos Health, 2006

Shelley Peterman Schwarz
Parkinson's Disease: 300 Tips for Making Life Easier, 2nd Edition
Demos Health, 2006

Daniel Stih
Healthy Living Spaces: Top 10 Hazards Affecting Your Health
Healthy Living Spaces, 2010

Vision and Hearing Resources

American Foundation for the Blind (Talking Books and Recorded Materials)
www.afb.org
800.232.5463

Braille Institute Accessibility Tools (customizing computer technology)
www.brailleinstitute.org/accessibility/

The Lighthouse Guild
www.lighthouseguild.org/programs-services/store
800.284.4422
05.0500
National Association of State Agencies for the Blind (specific state-by-state contacts)
www.ncsab.org

VisionAware: Resources for Independent Living with Vision Loss
www.visionaware.org

Service Animals

Assistance Dogs International (coalition of service dog organizations)
www.assistancedogsinternational.org

Canine Assistants
www.canineassistants.org/

Canine Companions for Independence
www.cci.org/

Dogs for Deaf and Disabled Americans
www.neads.org

Paws 4 Independence
www.paws4independence.com/

Paws with a Cause: Assistance Dogs
www.pawswithacause.org

SECTION EIGHT: SPECIAL SITUATIONS

MEMORY IMPAIRMENT

Memory impairment is heartbreaking.

So much of who we are and what we do is tied up in our memories: how to perform simple tasks; how to manage complex tasks; how to walk, run, skip, and turn cartwheels; how to recognize items and people; how to recall what happened in your childhood, throughout adulthood, and last week; how to remember what you had for dinner or where your car is parked or the name of the person you just ran into at the store.

We joke nervously about memory and "Old Timers Disease" as we age because certain elements of memory do seem to become more difficult for older people whether we're willing to admit it or not. There's also a bit of science to back up this observation. Names are harder to grab hold of or recall. Directions can seem more complicated. Future commitments and appointments need to be written down promptly. A T-shirt says it all: "I know I came into this room for a reason."

This is aging. It is not the same as brain damage, and brain damage of one sort or another is responsible for all memory impairment situations.

If you are dealing with memory impairment, a good place to start is with the Harvard Medical School Special Health Report on *Improving Memory,* which explores how memory works, changes with age, and can be impaired. If dementia is already fairly advanced, you may want to skip that and jump ahead to the Special Health Report called *A Guide to Alzheimer's Disease.*

People tend to think first of Alzheimer's and dementia when you mention memory impairment, which makes sense since over five million people have forms of dementia right now, a number that is projected to hit 7.1 million by 2025. But memory impairment can also be a component of numerous other medical problems.

Brain tumors and their treatment can really knock the hell out of what once was a nicely functioning organ. Strokes and cerebral hemorrhages disrupt normal blood flow through the brain, either by slowing it down with a clot or speeding it up with a leaking aneurysm, a weak patch in a blood vessel. Traumatic brain injuries can occur through accidents, warfare, or malice. Seizures send uncontrolled electrical currents pulsing through the brain. Infection is never good anywhere, but is exceptionally scary in the brain.

These are known as "events," a stunningly innocuous term considering the damage they cause. The aftermath of that damage varies because of countless factors, starting with the nature of the event, its location, and its duration.

Brain damage is sometimes reversible. Mostly it isn't.

The fact is that the brain is an extremely complicated and very delicate organ, and we don't know nearly as much about it as we would like to. We are now able to monitor many of the problems that occur inside the human skull, but aren't so good at preventing them.

While advances in imaging have made it possible to observe much more of what happens in the brain, this is a very well-protected organ and it's difficult to get a firsthand look. Neurosurgery is a serious endeavor that involves opening the cranium with power tools, then reaching the site of the problem by the shortest possible route. Cutting through *any* tissue encountered in the course of brain surgery has the potential to create major problems.

BRAIN TUMORS, STROKES, SEIZURES, AND BRAIN INJURIES

What all of these have in common is that they involve

sudden, life-altering changes to brain tissue—whether they make trouble immediately or hang out for a while before making a sudden and dramatic appearance. The TBIs (traumatic brain injuries) experienced by veterans of recent wars in the Middle East are a classic illustration that fits both models.

All of these have the potential to crash into a person's life with no warning. With almost all of them, you will probably have to deal with memory impairment. Depending on the nature of the brain event, this may or may not be permanent, and whether there are memory issues will probably be related to the wounded part of the brain.

The single most important book I have encountered for understanding these events and how to deal with their aftermath is *My Stroke of Insight* by Jill Bolte Taylor, who was using her doctorate in neuroanatomy at the Harvard Brain Bank (really!) when she experienced a massive stroke at the age of 37.

I only wish I'd had that book from the very beginning of my brother's stroke experiences. Her description of what the stroke felt like would have been invaluable to me—if for no other reason than it explained why my brother, a former police officer trained in emergency procedures, didn't call 911 after his own stroke. This failure to act baffled my sister and me, and almost certainly worsened his condition considerably.

Taylor's recovery from her stroke (actually a cerebral hemorrhage) was remarkable. It was also possible largely because her mother was able to devote herself to full-time caregiving and assistance with rehab, and because she herself worked relentlessly to recover.

The single most important part of *My Stroke of Insight* may be Appendix B, "Forty Things I Needed the Most." It's a caregiving and rehab blueprint that anybody dealing with brain problems can benefit from. Most of the forty items are specific requests for types of caregiving behavior that will benefit the patient and exercise the recovering brain: "Break all actions down into smaller steps of action." Others are more fundamental: "Love me for who I am today."

All are useful. I love this book.

My brother had memory problems, primarily short-term. This meant he had solid and accurate memories of the past, but wasn't able to retain new information about much of anything.

In his case, there was no single cause to blame, since he had the brain damage trifecta: a malignant brain tumor, a succession of major seizures over twelve years and, finally, strokes. (None of these actually killed him, as it happened. In that respect he was the Rasputin of Chicago.) He also had a history of taking his sweet time to get medical help for the seizures and strokes, and there were undoubtedly far more of both over time than he admitted—or, after a while, remembered.

This leads us to the absolute urgency for speed and calling for help when something goes awry.

The single most important thing anyone can do for a stroke or seizure is get help FAST. Indeed, the acronym FAST is used for on-the-spot diagnosis of possible strokes, and if you have any question about whether you or somebody else is experiencing a stroke, follow these steps:

- FACE—Can the person smile symmetrically, or is one side of the face drooping?
- ARMS—Can both arms be raised simultaneously and held upright?
- SPEECH—Can the person repeat a simple sentence clearly without slurring?
- TIME—If any of these tests go poorly, **CALL 911 IMMEDIATELY.**

The reason speed is so important is that certain clot-busting drugs can halt or even reverse some of the effects of a stroke, but they need to be administered within a few hours of the event. Wait too long and you lose that window of opportunity. While there are no comparable drugs for seizures, any seizure that lasts more than a few minutes needs professional evaluation and some major seizures simply won't stop on their own without medical intervention.

Either a stroke or a seizure can kill.

Rehab for strokes or other brain trauma often includes speech therapy, and how successful that is depends on the severity and location of the precipitating event. Understand that if memory impairment is also an issue, all rehab may be both difficult and lengthy.

ALL ALZHEIMER'S IS DEMENTIA, BUT ALL DEMENTIA IS NOT ALZHEIMER'S

Alzheimer's accounts for 60-80% of those diagnosed with dementia, with vascular dementia in some post-stroke patients the second most common form. However, a number of other forms of dementia manifest similar symptoms and challenges, and for the purposes of this discussion, we'll speak of all of these collectively as dementia.

Here's the official definition from the Alzheimer's Association website: *Dementia is a general term for a decline in mental ability severe enough to interfere with daily life.*

Whatever you call it, it's a growth industry. RAND Corporation estimates project that the cost of dementia care will double by 2040. Currently the Alzheimer's Association estimates that 2013 direct costs for Alzheimer's care will come to some $203 billion, including $142 billion for Medicare and Medicaid.

Alzheimer's is considered "early onset" if symptoms appear before age 65, though it may not be correctly diagnosed right away in a younger patient. Only about five percent of Alzheimer's patients are early onset, though that still adds up to 200,000 people in this disease of massive proportion.

A vast literature and many online resources cover every possible permutation of Alzheimer's, a word I don't remember ever hearing until I was well into adulthood, even though Herr Doktor Alzheimer identified it in Germany over a century ago in 1906—while San Francisco was on fire after the earthquake.

Back when we were kids, folks spoke of "premature

senility." We all knew pretty much what that meant: an older person who wasn't really *old,* but who was forgetful, confused, disoriented—and getting progressively worse on all fronts. There was also a kind of cultural understanding that *really* old people often couldn't remember things, except from long ago, and that senility was a normal part of the aging process.

Dementia has the potential to be a huge drain on baby boomers, many of whom have kept themselves in superb physical shape. This robust health insures that no other bodily system is particularly likely to conk out quickly.

Meanwhile we haven't seen a lot of developments in early diagnosis, treatment, medication, or reversal—despite some big research bucks and a clearly demonstrated market. A number of medications and treatments may slow down the disease or deal with particular behavioral situations, but that's as far as it goes.

PAPERWORK

Time is of the essence in getting paperwork signed by somebody who is moving into any form of dementia or is experiencing memory impairment.

You want to get your sibling on record about what she wants to do in terms of … well, everything. Start with the standard power of attorney since finances may have gotten into a muddle and bills will need to be paid. Then go for Advance Directives. And don't forget the Will.

If your sibling is extremely distressed and in denial, keep in mind that the paperwork isn't going to have "Alzheimer's" or "brain damage" splashed across it in red type. You can explain that this is critical information to have on record for *any* illness somebody might have. Which is true. If you've discussed these issues before, remind her of the conversation with as many details as you can come up with— place, time, who was there, other stuff going on at the same time. You can also point out that you and the other siblings are simultaneously completing the same types of paperwork for yourselves. In an ideal situation, this will also be perfectly true.

If your sibling is lucid and has already made her feelings known in writing about how she wants to proceed, you are very lucky.

If you wait too long, you may find yourself in court if family members are not in agreement. This is the last place you want to be at a time when everybody is already hideously stressed. The one glimmer of good news here is that if the patient's condition is that advanced, you will almost certainly have a diagnosis and medical recommendations for some form of enhanced care when you face the judge.

CAREGIVING AND DEMENTIA

By the time family members get involved with the care of a dementia patient, the disease is often quite advanced.

Since at this point there are no cures or significant preventive treatments, nobody can really be faulted for not seeking medical attention sooner. It's tough to blame your sister for pretending nothing was wrong, if that allowed her to delay the inevitable.

However, when a precipitating event brings the situation front and center, you may need to make some basic decisions really quickly.

The literature on dementia is extensive and its focus is overwhelmingly on caregiving. In addition to the Harvard Medical School's *A Guide to Alzheimer's Disease,* I'm also very impressed by *A Caregiver's Guide to Alzheimer's Disease: 300 Tips for Making Life Easier.* You may need to ration time to be able to even look at the relevant literature, however. I know a woman whose copy of *The Thirty-Six Hour Day,* a classic and time-honored dementia handbook, sat uncracked on her bedside table through the entire final year of her father's life.

Nearly every aspect of dementia caregiving differs from what we think of as traditional caregiving, since so frequently the patient is not otherwise ill. The Family Caregiver Alliance offers a superb Fact Sheet called "Caregiver's Guide to Understanding Dementia Behaviors" that will help you hit the ground upright, if not precisely running:

www.caregiver.org/caregivers-guide-understanding-dementia-behaviors.

Another useful online resource currently in development is "WeCare" which will help caregivers to understand, track, and treat neuropsychiatric symptoms (NPS). Part of the objective of this device is to ease some of the isolation experienced by dementia caregivers.

SUPPORT GROUPS

You need at least one support group when dealing with dementia or severe memory impairment, and I recommend having a couple: one online, one in person. There's more information on these in the chapter on "Caregiving."

While you may not realize it immediately, it also helps people in support groups to be able to give assistance to somebody else. Paying it forward can feel rewarding when your own situation may not be so great.

SAFETY CONSIDERATIONS

One of the toughest responsibilities for memory impairment caregiving is assuring the safety of the patient.

This can require the same kind of vigilance that is necessary with toddlers and varies on a case-by-case basis. One person may be prone to wandering off, another to leaving stove burners blazing, a third to falling for scammers and telephone solicitors. You need to figure out what the safety threats are to your sibling and act accordingly.

If somebody is prone to wandering away, you need to be proactive. My friend Lenore and her Search-and-Rescue dog Karma are prepared to head out looking for your missing brother, but it's a lot easier all around if their services aren't necessary.

Start by making it a little harder to get outside, or into problem areas like the basement. (If you are securing exits, of course, this obviously requires that somebody be around in case of fire.) Simple slide bolts at the top or bottom of a door may be all it takes. You can also get electronically controlled lock systems.

If you aren't on the scene and the object of your concern is living alone, one excellent safeguard is the Safe Return program run by the Alzheimer's Association in conjunction with MedicAlert.

MedicAlert is a smart idea for anybody with a serious health problem, since paramedics automatically look for the distinctive (but reasonably discreet) jewelry that signals registration and ongoing medical issues. At that point, responders contact MedicAlert via an 800 number to determine the patient's medical problem and learn about medications that might interfere with or complicate emergency services. A caregiver can get matched registration so that if something happens to her, MedicAlert will know who to contact to care for the suddenly-stranded patient. www.alz.org/care/dementia-medic-alert-safe-return.asp

Newer technology offers more sophisticated possibilities, including Comfort Zone, which uses a form of GPS tracking to keep an eye on The Wanderer and report when he goes beyond a physical area predetermined by the subscriber. A related Comfort Zone check-in service provides on-demand location checks. www.alz.org/comfortzone/

Meanwhile back at the ranch, keep an eye on what's in the refrigerator or left out overnight on the counter. Pitch anything that is getting funky or has a sell-by-date from last year. Your sister has enough problems without adding food poisoning to the list.

Get a spare pair of eyeglasses or dentures and monitor the administration and timing of medications. Take a peek at trash cans before you dump them to be sure nothing ended up in there by mistake.

Make sure the batteries are fresh in all smoke detectors.

DRIVING AND
MEMORY IMPAIRMENT

Driving is equivalent to independence in modern American society, and we've all heard stories about how hard it is to take car keys taken away from parents unwilling to lose this freedom.

Most of these are situations where vision problems, infirmity, or slow reflexes are the primary concern. Memory impairment brings in such other critical factors as spatial perception and planning, not to mention distractibility.

If you think it's difficult taking car keys away from a septuagenarian, octogenarian or nonagenarian, you are correct. But it's a whole lot tougher with somebody younger. The sister who taught you how to drive, for example, or the brother who sometimes let you borrow his car for a really big date.

It can be done, however. I say that as somebody who orchestrated taking away a truck and its keys from a 51-year-old ex-cop and lived to tell the tale, albeit at a distance. I had a great support team for this, fortunately, and you'll want to bring out your own top players if you expect a lot of trouble.

Unless your sibling initiates the conversation about this situation, expect a lot of trouble.

If the thought of riding shotgun with your brother gives you the willies, it's time to take action. You don't want to wait until something terrible happens. He may be only planning to drive down the hill to the grocery store, but if he gets distracted or disoriented and plows into a bunch of school kids waiting at a bus stop, it will be far too late.

By all means blame the decision on the doctor if it will help. If the doc didn't bring the subject up in the first place, it's a pretty safe bet that she will back the no-driving decision enthusiastically, quite possibly in writing. If she won't and you're sure your brother has no business behind the wheel, you may want to think about finding another doctor.

The Mayo Clinic Guide to Alzheimer's Disease has an excellent section on "Travel and Safety" which covers a lot of things I'd never thought of. These include some sneaky ways to get around the issue. Hide the car and say it's in the shop, for instance. Have a mechanic install a kill switch. Or substitute a set of keys that look right but don't work.

ALTERNATE TRANSPORTATION

There are plenty of alternative ways of getting around, with or without dementia. Work these out before you grab the keys.

Is there a local senior shuttle service of some sort? A group from your brother's church that takes shut-ins to the grocery store or shops for them? Does the local medical center have a van or ambulette service?

This may even be covered by insurance for medical appointments or therapy sessions. My brother's shuttle to rehab after his first stroke was covered by his policy, and driven by a retired cop from his own police department, to boot. (He still hated it.)

Maybe your brother lives in an area with excellent bus, rail, and subway service. If that's the case, he's probably already accustomed to using public transit. Figure out the regular routes he'll need, get to know them, and ride along with him as a test. If he is likely to be using a particular route at a regular time, it can't hurt to get friendly with the bus driver, too.

Rural areas may offer other kinds of services. The Southern Illinois county where my brother spent his final year had an excellent free van service that would pick up seniors or the disabled at home and deliver them to doctor appointments and other obligations.

Finally, there are usually people who handle transportation for seniors at whatever level and frequency is required, often on an appointment basis.

Like *Driving Miss Daisy,* except that Morgan Freeman probably isn't available.

ORGANIZING FOR
MEMORY IMPAIRMENT

Whether you are setting up systems for someone with newly acquired memory problems from a stroke or brain-related illness or you're looking down the road to simplify matters for a dementia patient, the basic principles remain the same.

If your sibling is still living independently, you'll want to build in as many crutches as possible to continue that independence: labels, items grouped together where she expects to find them, reminders to take medication posted prominently (along with alarms or other audio reminders at meds time), handrails on stairs, and grab bars in bathtubs.

Think along the same lines as when you were childproofing your own home to protect toddlers.

Keep the modifications appropriate to the person, however. There's no point in removing a doorknob to keep a lifelong handyman from leaving a room if he can grab a couple of paper clips and get the door open in seventeen seconds.

Try to keep an eye on functionality and make things as simple as you can without losing the familiarity that makes your sister want to stay in her home in the first place. Get rid of the throw rugs and trailing cords, rearrange furniture to minimize obstacles, and widen pathways. Plug in nightlights all over the place, and make sure the path between bedroom and bathroom is lit up like an airport runway.

If stairs are an issue, think about setting up a downstairs bedroom, and call it temporary if your sister sees this as a loss of autonomy. If her home is cluttered with photos and objets d'art (or objets d'kitsch) remove or at least box up some of the excess. If she notices, tell her you're rotating things. Then try to remember to rotate them, unless she doesn't mention it again, in which case that task is done.

Store similar objects together, and do it in a place that she associates with those things. If she is already confused, it will only complicate matters if you put all her socks in a different drawer. Keep like with like: keys on a single rack hanging by the back door; coffee, mug, and creamer in the cupboard by the coffee maker; sweaters, coats, and boots in a hall closet.

A single logical spot where frequently-used items live is a good idea for anybody, and especially useful with memory impairment.

If you make that spot obvious and visible—a shelf or table near the door is perfect—the transition to that new system will be smoother. Here's where keys, wallet, purse, cell phone, sunglasses, reading glasses, flashlight, and gloves can live. A basket or bowl works fine for the little stuff.

This is not the time for bright new ideas on efficiently using space. You may believe that extra paper products belong in the linen closet, but if they've always lived in the basement or the garage, that's where your sister is going to look for a new roll of paper towels. And storing rarely-used serving platters in the oven won't seem like such a great idea when she turns on the broiler one day and they all break.

If it will cause too much stress to get rid of excess similar items, push the fourteen infrequently-used saucepans to the back of the cabinet and leave her favorite two up front.

Keep things in sight when it's possible. If she wants to keep the pot she uses every day on the stove and is conscientious about turning off burners, leave it there. Frequently-used kitchen items can hang from hooks or be visible in a jar by the stove. And don't forget Velcro, which can be stuck to almost anything to give it a permanent and easily-seen home.

Labels are hugely helpful, and label makers are cheap and readily available. Make those labels as large as vision problems dictate, but in general they can be pretty unobtrusive. Clear label tape is even more subdued. I placed discreet labels on the bottom corners of my brother's kitchen cabinets and all his office drawers. They worked just fine and weren't obnoxious.

For a person having difficulty reading, you can easily substitute pictures for labels. Use a digital camera to photograph the contents of a cabinet or to identify the pair of shoes in each box on your sister's closet shelf. In a pinch, cut pictures out of magazines.

If somebody can't remember where something is without seeing it, consider removing cabinet doors. This is particularly helpful in the kitchen or bathroom.

You're not aiming for a spread in a decorating magazine here. You're trying to make life easier for your sibling—and by extension for everybody else.

THE NEW ART OF CONVERSATION

In my experience, there are three different kinds of conversational issues where brain problems are concerned. The first is difficulty finding the appropriate words and/or getting those words from the brain to the tongue.

My brother suffered from this, and "suffer" is a very relevant verb for man who was once spectacularly articulate. Because he started out with an extensive vocabulary he was frequently able to substitute synonyms when the words he wanted wouldn't come, but he still hated it and hated even more that we could figure out what he was doing.

I wouldn't even want to guess how many hundreds of times he said, "I know what I want to say, but I can't get the words from here"—pointing to his brain—"to here"—pointing to his tongue. It was tough on all of us, and as he became weaker over time this obligatory introduction would sometimes wear him out so much that he never did get around to what he had been trying/hoping to say.

A variant of this situation is when the word that does come out is totally wrong and obviously not what your sibling had in mind. This is embarrassing on both ends, and if you can find a way to make light of it, you'll both be ahead of the game.

Sometimes it can be useful to offer prompts or suggestions, though some people find that even more frustrating than being unable to produce the word correctly in the first place. Also, if you start guessing and get it wrong, you can end up with a game of "find that word" that everybody hates, a hideous verbal edition of Charades.

I sometimes had to remind myself to tell my brother that I understood how frustrating he found this speech problem, but it helped us both when I was able to. Plus, I came to realize, he didn't remember all the other times I'd told him the same thing anyway, because his short-term memory was also fried.

Patience is your friend. For some of us, patience does not come easily.

The second conversational roadblock is short-term memory problems.

Here an event or conversation occurs, but the brain's mechanism for processing and cataloguing it is broken. Sheer force of repetition may help with something important like: *Never leave the kitchen when a burner is turned on.* Visual reminders of important issues can also be useful.

When short-term memory is a problem, it can help to begin a conversation by making a general statement that gets some facts on the table right away, before confusion starts to set in. "We talked last night about going to the grocery store today" is better than "Are you ready to go?" Where? When? For what?

Do your best to not get annoyed or be patronizing. Try to always remember that this is much harder on the person who is desperately trying to communicate. And if you can possibly avoid it, don't say things like "Don't you remember what I said yesterday about that?" or "I've told you that a hundred times."

Keep in mind that this is a more evil cousin of the same general situation that we all experience. You reach the garage, can't recall why you headed there in the first place, and have to go back to where you started the journey to remember that you need a screwdriver.

The difference is that for short-term memory loss, going back to a starting point won't help retrieve information that never got catalogued and stored in the first place.

The final conversational problem area is with full-on dementia. Dementia patients frequently have short-term memory problems, but that's the tip of the memory iceberg. They may also believe that it is a different era altogether— perhaps one when they were employed, newlywed, or spending summer at the childhood beach house.

Once upon a time, people believed that it was necessary to keep the dementia patient firmly grounded in reality, even if this meant continual reminders that a beloved husband was dead for six years and that you were her daughter and not her Aunt Edna. Today's kinder, gentler philosophy allows for the use of little white lies to comfort both caregiver and patient.

Once again, patience is crucial. There's no point in speaking more loudly unless there's a concurrent hearing problem, though you may need to repeat things many times— preferably without saying, "I just *told* you that" or "Weren't you paying attention?" or "How many times do I need to remind you?"

Pay attention to particular problem areas and use simpler language if that helps. Avoid open-ended questions, particularly if they require specific answers. "Do you want to watch TV?" is better than "What TV program should we watch?"

Inside Alzheimer's by Nancy Pearce is full of warm and caring information and anecdotes about communicating with loved ones suffering from dementia, and *Talking to Alzheimer's* by Claudia J. Strauss has plenty of very specific ideas on what to say and what not to say.

And if you want the real inside story, Lisa Snyder has taped conversations with seven dementia patients in *Speaking Our Minds: Personal Reflections from Individuals with Alzheimer's.*

They will break your heart.

ADDITIONAL INFORMATION

Alzheimer's Disease and Dementia

Alzheimer's Foundation of America
www.alzfdn.org/
866.232.8484

Alzheimer's Association
www.alz.org/
800.272.3900

Association for Frontotemporal Degeneration
http://www.theaftd.org
866.507.7222

Caregiver's Guide to Understanding Dementia Behaviors
www.caregiver.org/caregivers-guide-understanding-dementia-behaviors

• • • • •

Naheed Ali
Understanding Alzheimer's
Rowman & Littlefield, 2012

Marjorie Allen, Susan Dublin, Patricia Kimmerly
A Look Inside Alzheimer's
Demos Health, 2012

P. Murali Doraiswamy and Lisa P. Wyther, with Tina Adler
The Alzheimer's Action Plan: What You Need to Know—and What You Can Do—About Memory Problems, from Prevention to Early Intervention and Care
St. Martin's, 2009

Harvard Medical School Special Health Reports
A Guide to Alzheimer's Disease
Harvard Medical School, 2012

Ronald Petersen
Mayo Clinic Guide to Alzheimer's Disease
Mayo Clinic, 2006

Lisa Snyder
Speaking Our Minds: Personal Reflections from Individuals with Alzheimer's
W.H. Freeman & Co., 1999

Amy L. Sutton, ed.
Alzheimer Disease Sourcebook, 5th Edition
Omnigraphics Health Reference Series, 2011

Brain Tumors

American Brain Tumor Association
www.abta.org   800.886.2282

National Brain Tumor Society
www.braintumor.org/

Peter Black
Living with a Brain Tumor: Dr. Peter Black's Guide to Taking Control of Your Treatment
Holt, 2006

Deanna Glass Macenka and Alessandro Olivi
Johns Hopkins Patients' Guide to Brain Cancer
Jones and Bartlett, 2011

John W. Kerastas
Chief Complaint: Brain Tumor
Sunstone Press, 2012

Virginia Stark-Vance and Mary Louise Dubay
100 Questions and Answers About Brain Tumors, 2nd Edition
Jones and Bartlett Publishers, 2010

Lynne P. Taylor, Alyx B. Porter Umphrey, and Diane Richard
Navigating Life with a Brain Tumor
Oxford University Press, 2012

Tim B. Ward
Surviving and Thriving: A Brain Tumor Survivor's Story
Outskirts Press, 2010

Brain Injury

John W. Cassidy
Mindstorms: The Complete Guide for Families Living with Traumatic Brain Injury
Da Capo Press, 2009

Carolyn E. Dolen
Brain Injury Rewiring for Loved Ones
Idyll Arbor, 2010

Rahul Jandial
100 Questions & Answers About Head and Brain Injuries
Jones and Bartlett, 2009

Michael Paul Mason
Head Cases: Stories of Brain Injury and Its Aftermath
Farrar, Strauss & Giroux, 2008

Cheryle Sullivan
Brain Injury Survival Kit: 365 Tips, Tools & Tricks to Deal with Cognitive Function Loss
Demos Health, 2008

Memory Impairment and Caregiving

Anne Davis Basting
Forget Memory: Creating Better Lives for People with Dementia
Johns Hopkins Press, 2009

Patricia Callone and Connie Kudlacek
The Alzheimer's Caregiving Puzzle: Putting Together the Pieces
Demos Health, 2010

Patricia R. Callone, Connie Kudlacek, Barbara C. Vasiloff,
Janaan Manternach, and Roger A. Brumback
A Caregiver's Guide to Alzheimer's Disease: 300 Tips for Making Life Easier
Demos Medical Publishing, 2006

Harvard Medical School Special Health Reports
Improving Memory: Understanding Age-Related Memory Loss
Harvard Medical School, 2012

Nancy L. Mace and Peter V. Rabins
The 36 Hour Day: A Family Guide to Caring for People with Alzheimer Disease, Related Dementias, and Memory Loss, 5th Edition
Johns Hopkins Press, 2011

Maria M. Meyer and Paula Derr
The Comfort of Home for Alzheimer's Disease: A Guide for Caregivers
Care Trust Publications, 2007

Nancy Pearce
Inside Alzheimer's: How to Hear and Honor Connections with a Person Who Has Dementia
Forasson Press, 2007

Lisa Radin and Gary Radin
What if it's Not Alzheimer's? A Caregiver's Guide to Dementia
Prometheus Books, 2008

Mark Warner
The Complete Guide to Alzheimer's Proofing Your Home
Purdue University Press, 2000

Laura Wayman
A Loving Approach to Dementia Care: Making Meaningful Connections with the Person Who Has Alzheimer's Disease or Other Dementia or Memory Loss
Johns Hopkins Press, 2011

Helen Buell Whitworth and James A. Whitworth
A Caregiver's Guide to Lewy Body Dementia
Demos Health, 2010

Vaughan E. James
The Alzheimer's Advisor: A Caregiver's Guide to Dealing with the Tough Legal and Practical Issues
Amacon, 2009

Stroke

American Stroke Association
www.strokeassociation.org
888.4.STROKE

National Stroke Association
www.stroke.org
1.800.STROKES

Stroke Network
www.stroke-network.com/

Kinan K. Hreib
100 Questions & Answers About Stroke: A Lahey Clinic Guide
Jones and Bartlett, 2009

Cleo Hutton
After a Stroke: 300 Tips for Making Life Easier
Demos Health, 2005

Peter G. Levine
Stronger After Stroke, 2nd Edition
Demos Health, 2012

Maria M. Meyer
The Comfort of Home for Stroke: A Guide for Caregivers
CareTrust Publications, 2007

Jill Bolte Taylor
My Stroke of Insight: A Brain Scientist's Personal Journey
Viking, 2008

SIBLINGS DISABLED
FROM BIRTH

Most of us involved in the care of ailing siblings come late to the party, showing up to try to help somebody on the sunset side of adulthood. Our brothers and sisters are mostly coping with the kind of illnesses you contract when you can no longer call yourself middle-aged with a straight face.

Matters are very different for those whose families include what we now call special needs children. And whether that means the revelation of Down Syndrome before or at birth or a constellation of unfolding symptoms in infancy and childhood which may be diagnosed, rediagnosed, and misdiagnosed indefinitely, it changes the dynamic of a family.

Any family.

In most cases this is because the special needs child requires additional time and attention from the parents, whose marriage may also be challenged by an unanticipated—and face it, unwelcome—change in the way everybody had assumed family life was going to go. Often the special needs child has severe medical issues of some sort, requiring a whole new level of parental advocacy. This whole familial stew is then seasoned with varying amounts of guilt, confusion, and resentment—and shaken daily.

WHEN YOU HAVE A
SIBLING DISABLED FROM BIRTH

If you have a sibling disabled from birth, the environment in which you grow up will initially seem to be normal—because for your family, it is.

And then over time you will begin to notice that your world seems a little bit ... different. Because it is. If you are an older sib, the chronology differs a bit and you may see things go south in a hurry when a baby sister or brother with disabilities is born.

While you're growing up you may not realize, or be able to acknowledge, how thoroughly your life is intertwined with the fortunes and misfortunes of your sibling. Some of this intertwining may also complicate your own life, restrict your own activities and options, and require too much maturity too soon.

You have probably felt embarrassed—and ashamed to be embarrassed. Guilt-plagued in general. You may have been mortified in public places by sibling outbursts or tantrums, or watched your family torn to pieces by life-altering heartaches and medical crises and impossible responsibilities.

It's likely that you've advocated for your disabled sibling, perhaps against your own parents. Most of all, over the years, you are forced far too often into tough, no-win choices: sibling versus spouse, battles with bureaucracies that shift and misclassify, reluctant placements into living situations which are far from ideal.

And you always live with an awareness that one day the responsibility for your sibling is likely to transfer to you.

When that happens, whatever living situation is in place for your brother or sister may change. In fact, it's almost certain to, whether your sib lives with your aging parents, in a group home, in semi-independence, or in some sort of institution.

One day you will have to do *something,* even if it's just flee on a guilt-slicked downhill track reminiscent of an Olympic luge course.

SUPPORT GROUPS

Nobody dealing with a sibling's health issues could be described as lucky, but for people on the challenging journey of life with a disabled sibling, there's one shining beacon.

An informed, intelligent, and compassionate community is already in place and you can step right into it.

The Sibling Support Network and Sibling Leadership Network both exist to work with and advocate for siblings of men and women with profound physical and mental disabilities.

You don't have to explain how you feel or apologize for anything. These people really *do* know what you're thinking and why, and how your life has gone and where it's likely to be headed. They've been on that same road themselves. They are warm and welcoming, sharing all kinds of practical information and resources.

In the years since I first attached myself to the periphery of these groups, I have watched time and time again as somebody discovers them and collapses into the cushioning welcome of people who understand exactly what they are going through because they've been there themselves.

Early on during my experiences with my brother's illness, I began looking online for resources on dealing with ailing siblings. I found almost nothing, and clung for dear life to a Yahoo Groups list called SibNet. For me it was a lifesaver.

This list has a thousand members and its more active sister group on Facebook has 2,500. You need to apply to become a member and participate, in order to protect everybody's privacy. Only siblings are allowed: no parents, children, friends, researchers, or trolls.

Both are components of the Sibling Support Network. The SibNet lists (there are others for kids, teens, and grandparents) grew out of SibShops, workshops for children growing up with disabled brothers and sisters.

SibShops were the brainchild of Don Meyer, a Seattle psychologist with two hearing-impaired brothers. In less than twenty years, over 400 SibShops have been created in eight countries, and training sessions are held every year, both in the US and abroad.

The Sibling Survival Guide was written by members of these communities and edited by Don Meyer and Emily Holl. It is incredible.

The Sibling Survival Guide is focused on adults with developmental disabilities, but it covers plenty of territory and addresses just about every situation that a sibling of an adult with any kind of disabilities is likely to confront. It moves gracefully from social situations to research protocols to legal intricacies that most people never have to think about.

It forms an excellent companion volume to an earlier book of personal accounts by many of the same participants. *Thicker Than Water* illustrates how the processes and particulars of integrating a special needs child into the family have varied over time and around the world.

The successes and the supportiveness of these groups offer a splendid example of how siblings can assist one another with advice, resources, suggestions, and a way to vent about their particular problems in safe and controlled settings.

What to do? When to do it? How to deal with elderly parents in denial and other siblings who checked out of the family situation one way or another? And what about the sibs themselves, likely to outlive their frequently overprotective parents and land in the spare bedrooms of fearful and often unprepared adult brothers and sisters?

The SibNet participants I've been watching all these years span at least six decades, and form a family all their own. They live all around the world, the occasional post from Italy or Japan or Israel a reminder that these situations occur everywhere. Some disabled siblings have passed away, and their survivors grieve with a special, focused intensity. Other list members are young, looking out at uncertain adulthood with an awareness beyond any denial that at some point everything can and will change dramatically, and probably not when they're expecting it, or ready.

As if anyone is ever ready. For any of it.

I found a shorthand here, an undercurrent of commonality that makes the best internet lists so useful and nurturing and informative. So can you.

ADDITIONAL INFORMATION

AAIDD: American Association on Intellectual and
Developmental Disabilities   www.aamr.org/

The Arc: For People with Intellectual and Developmental
Disabilities   www.thearc.org/ 800.433.5255

AUCD: Association of University Centers on Disabilities
www.aucd.org/

Autism Society
www.autism-society.org/

NACDD: National Association of Councils on Developmental
Disabilities
www.nacdd.org

NADD: An Association for Persons with Developmental
Disabilities and Mental Health Needs
www.thenadd.org/

SABE USA: Self Advocates Becoming Empowered
www.sabeusa.org/

Sibling Leadership Network
www.siblingleadership.org/

Sibling Support Network (SibNet and SibNet on Facebook)
www.siblingsupport.org/

Source America: Creating Employment Opportunities for
People with Significant Disabilities
www.sourceamerica.org/

United Cerebral Palsy
www.ucp.org/

• • • • •

Terrell Harris Dougan
That Went Well: Adventures in Caring for My Sister
Hyperion, 2009

Eileen Garvin
How to Be a Sister: A Love Story with a Twist of Autism
The Experiment, 2010

Paul Karasik and Judy Karasik
The Ride Together: A Brother and Sister's Memoir of Autism in the Family
Washington Square Press, 2003

Don Meyer, ed.
Thicker Than Water: Essays by Adult Siblings of People with Disabilities
Woodbine House, 2009

Don Meyer and Emily Holl, editors
The Sibling Survival Guide
Woodbine House, 2014

Mary McHugh
Special Siblings: Growing Up with Someone with a Disability
Paul H. Brookes Publishing, 2002

Susan Meyers
Check This Box if You Are Blind: A Brother, A Sister, A True Story
Climbing Ivy Press, 2011

Jean Safer
The Normal One: Life with a Difficult or Damaged Sibling
Delta, 2003

Rachel Simon
Riding the Bus with My Sister: A True Life Journey
Houghton Mifflin Harcourt, 2002

Kate Strohm
Being the Other One: Growing Up with a Brother or Sister who has Special Needs
Shambhala, 2005

MENTAL ILLNESS AND SUBSTANCE ABUSE

Mental illness and substance abuse are discussed together here not because they are related problems or subsets of one another, though this may sometimes be the case. It's because there are so many similarities in how these problems manifest themselves and affect not only the person in question, but all those in the surrounding area.

If that area includes your family gene pool, you already know the inherent problems. You may have been living in their shadow for most of your life, and you may also have personal experience with mental illness or addiction or both.

STIGMA

Let's get this out in the open right away.

Mental illness and substance abuse both carry stigmas. It shouldn't be that way, but it is. How deep or pervasive those stigmas are is often a product of the community or region in which you live. So is the likelihood of finding boots-on-the-ground help. The reality is that you are more likely to find knowledgeable local resources for either in San Francisco or New York than in the Upper Midwest or the rural Bible Belt.

Knowing when and how to swallow your pride and seek help can be nearly as rough for those around the ailing or addicted person as it is for the actual victim. "Victim" begs the question as well, since a mature and intelligent discussion of either mental illness or substance abuse all but demands that the person with an illness or addiction be regarded as a patient with a disease. This has nothing to do with being politically correct, either. It's a matter of medical reality.

Meanwhile, people who act in societally-inappropriate ways because of substance abuse or mental illness often appear to be everywhere.

And sometimes they are related to you, more closely than may feel comfortable.

DENIAL

There's also a huge Catch-22 in both mental illness and substance abuse cases: The illness itself may inform the patient that there really isn't anything wrong.

This is particularly pernicious in instances of mental illness, but anyone who has ever grappled with addiction—whether first- or second-hand—will recognize the internal voice saying, "Don't worry what they say. It's their problem if they don't like it. You're just fine."

Be aware that you may not be able to do anything to help or improve your sibling's condition if that voice is louder than yours.

MENTAL ILLNESS AND SUBSTANCE ABUSE: THEN AND NOW

People didn't used to talk about mental illness or substance abuse. Both tended to be regarded as evidence of personal failure and lack of moral substance.

Somebody might be said to feel down in the dumps or to have a bit of a drinking problem, but nobody was tossing around words like clinical depression or alcoholism. Folks who wouldn't dream of telling a friend or relative with cancer to just suck it up and recover didn't hesitate to assume that the depressed would cheer up if you reminded them frequently enough to smile, or that out-of-control drinking was a character defect and not a function of biochemistry.

While the medical and scientific evidence to the contrary has advanced dramatically, the revised line of thinking hasn't always kept pace among the general public.

PSYCHOLOGIST VS. PSYCHIATRIST

Psychiatrists are physicians who have completed medical school and extensive additional training. They are licensed by the states where they practice and can prescribe medications.

Psychologists are not medical doctors, though many have doctorate degrees, and are also licensed by the states where they practice. They are not able to write prescriptions, but often work in conjunction with doctors who can.

Psychologists deal with a wide range of everyday problems as well as with mental illness and may specialize in such areas as couples counseling, troubled teens, drug rehab, PTSD, or just about any type of problem you can think of. If you're dealing with a very specific mental health problem, you'll save time and money if you look for a psychologist specializing in that area before diving into treatment.

TALK THERAPY

Conventional wisdom changes all the time, which is why it isn't simply called wisdom.

One area that illustrates this point is talk therapy, which can be useful for all sorts of short-term problems. You don't always need to seek professional help to use it, either. That's what friends are for, and women are much better at this than men. However, if you're looking for a professional to talk to, you're more likely to end up with a psychologist than a psychiatrist, a distinction which also has to do with billing rates.

Be aware, however, that talk therapy is generally fairly useless with mental illness, unless in conjunction with some form of cognitive behavioral therapy and/or medication. One reason for this is that so many forms of mental illness feature a small insistent internal voice claiming that shrinks are all a load of crap, there's no problem anyway, and everything is really just fine.

PSYCHIATRIC MEDS

Psychiatric medication first was introduced in the mid-20th Century when Thorazine came to market in 1950. Modern chemistry and pharmacology have been going gangbusters ever since, to the extent that Wikipedia now lists six categories:
- Antidepressants
- Stimulants
- Antipsychotics
- Mood stabilizers
- Anxiolytics
- Depressants
- Psychedelics

Each of these categories has subcategories and those are often further subdivided. Try not to overthink or over-research this, and keep in mind that the brain is the least-well-understood body organ by a huge margin. The best approach when somebody is prescribed psychiatric meds is to ask a lot of questions, research the specific medication, and try not to panic if its primary use is something that you didn't even think was a problem.

I once went into a cold research frenzy when my unhappy brother, who was staying 1,800 miles from his home with my sister, was prescribed a drug that I quickly learned was considered an antipsychotic. He's *not* psychotic, I wanted to scream from the rooftop, he's just frustrated and he wants to go home.

But the medication helped in what was rapidly becoming a crisis situation, and it helped almost instantly. Later when he was living in a different setting, it was possible to discontinue the drug, and we did so.

Here's the lesson I took away from this. If you are wrestling with psychiatric medications on behalf of any loved one, including yourself, you ought to make it a mantra:

The only thing that matters is that it is working right now.

It used to be that if you became severely depressed, about all you could do about it was go to a mental hospital and make potholders. Eventually, it was hoped, you'd cheer up again and go home.

People are still sometimes hospitalized for depression or other mental illnesses, but the first line of defense today is almost always pharmacological.

The most commonly prescribed psychiatric meds in the early 21st Century are antidepressants, suggestive of a massive societal minefield that we are going to simply tiptoe around during this discussion. Big Pharma has been working hard on this category of drugs and they've come up with some excellent medications, particularly in the SSRI (selective serotonin reuptake inhibitor) subcategory.

It sometimes seems as if everyone in town is taking antidepressants for one thing or another. This is perhaps not surprising when you consider that antidepressants are now commonly prescribed for depression, bulimia, generalized anxiety disorder (GAD), panic disorder, post-traumatic stress disorder (PTSD), obsessive-compulsive disorder (OCD), and social anxiety disorder. They are also used off-label for numerous other ailments, and in conjunction with medications that treat other problems. Oncology patients often are prescribed antidepressants since it is unquestionably depressing to have cancer.

Antidepressants can be particularly helpful for people going through unusually rocky periods, and many people use them for a while—then stop and never look back.

Are antidepressants overprescribed? Probably. Does that matter in your family's specific case? Probably not.

To the extent that antidepressants help somebody deal with a difficult medical condition, they are invaluable. It is possible to see a loved one (or oneself) improve almost overnight with the right medication, and these are *Hallelujah!* moments.

However, people are sensitive to all medications in different ways, and what works for one person may be a disaster for another. Sometimes it can also take a while to find the proper medication or medication combo, and in some instances it's necessary to try more than one possibility—each for weeks on end while waiting for relief that doesn't come. This is enormously discouraging and a lot of people give up at this point, when they may be one prescription away from genuine relief.

Side-effects can range from minimal to crippling, and an individual has to decide whether the good outweighs the bad in some of these cases. Weight gain is a common side-effect from many psychiatric meds. In that instance, a friend once said simply, "I decided it was better to be fat and happy than thin and miserable."

Also, you may not be able to count on this successful chemical cocktail being a permanent solution. Sometimes psychiatric meds stop working after a while for no obvious reason—they get bored, they want to go to Paris, who knows?—and you have to go through the whole process again.

As with any medication, pay close attention to what is being prescribed and how it is to be taken. If something is supposed to be taken at a particular time or day, ask why. Does food taken at the same time make things better or worse? Ask about potential side-effects and if there are similar medications to try if a particular one doesn't work out.

It is customary to start out with lower dosages of these meds and see how the patient tolerates them before increasing the dosage. If things go well, congratulate yourself and the patient and keep the next appointment for any necessary changes or increases in dosage. If things go badly, contact the doctor's office immediately for instructions.

Watch out for potentially troublesome interactions with alcohol or recreational drugs, especially if you're dealing with somebody who has a history of using or abusing either. You'll probably have to look online to check on interactions with recreational drugs. Physicians often lump all recreational drugs together under the heading of Horrible Things—as does the DEA, which classifies both heroin and marijuana as Class I drugs, the category considered most dangerous.

HOMEOPATHIC MEDICATION
IS STILL MEDICATION

People who are accustomed to using supplements and homeopathic medications often want to apply this technique to mental health problems. This approach sometimes is very successful, but it can also create real problems.

First, it may not work.

Second, most supplements and herbal remedies are not subject to FDA testing or specific standards of strength. So somebody taking St. John's Wort for depression, say, could buy five different brands at the same health food store and then be in possession of five very different dosages, even if the labels claim they are the same strength.

Third, and perhaps most important, when somebody who's been using these remedies does agree to try 21st Century pharmacology, it must be an either-or situation. It's tricky enough to determine and monitor dosages of psychiatric meds without adding holistic wild cards.

CAN YOU COMMIT SOMEBODY
WITHOUT CONSENT?

"I'll have you committed."

It's a grand threat and one that anybody dealing with serious mental illness has articulated at least in the privacy of the shower. Unfortunately, the public reality is a lot more complicated and generally requires the consent of the person involved.

In general, you can't simply have somebody committed because you know it's the appropriate action. There are all kinds of requirements, many a function of state and local law. If this is something that you are seriously considering, safety issues may be a factor, but in order to protect patient rights, there are still likely to be a lot of hoops to jump through.

And even if you are able to have somebody committed—after a very public demonstration of inappropriate behavior, for example—it is generally for a limited period of time and subject to judicial review.

Your best bet to answer this question is to consult local law enforcement, mental health, and/or medical authorities. Prepare to be frustrated and quite possibly disappointed by the answers they give you.

GOING OFF THEIR MEDS

We hear the phrase so often that it's become a cliché, but the reality is that people who have been prescribed psychiatric medications often don't like taking them.

This may be because of side-effects, or expense, or denial, or because the meds blunt elements of a mental illness which the patient doesn't mind at all. Bipolar patients, for instance, may take medication to control both manic and depressive stages, but many people enjoy the good feelings and increased productivity of a manic phase and hate to lose it.

Sometimes if meds are very effective, people become convinced they aren't necessary.

If you are dealing with somebody who routinely goes off prescribed medication, the best approach is to try to determine why—in as nonjudgmental fashion as possible. From there you can attempt to find a solution, working with the patient and doctor. There may be a different medication which would work better, for instance, or a more appropriate dosage. It's always worth asking.

Just don't expect it to be easy.

SELF-MEDICATION

Patients with mental illness are notorious for attempts to self-medicate in order to make unwanted symptoms go away.

This may involve the use of alcohol or illegal drugs, and it can make matters very difficult for a sibling who's trying to help the patient move forward on more traditional treatment paths.

SUBSTANCE USE VERSUS SUBSTANCE ABUSE

One issue which makes it difficult to deal with substance abuse is that our society doesn't officially differentiate between using a substance and abusing it.

By comparison, lots of people drink alcohol without having problems. We see them everywhere: on television, in bars, in our own homes. Most are what we call social drinkers.

We do not identify social drug users as being equally harmless, however, and substance abuse is an area where simple possession of many materials is not only illegal, but punishable by major incarceration.

So what do we know about use versus abuse? Very little. For starters, smart people are not inclined to announce that they use controlled substances with no ill effects. This may be because of denial. But it is more likely to mean that the person in question doesn't want to make a pointless stand and get arrested.

The assumption that use equals abuse needs to be addressed, but the only arena in which that is happening at all is in the realm of marijuana, which didn't reach its tipping point across the nation until recreational marijuana was approved by voters in Colorado and Washington. This occurred in 2014, eighteen years after California voters passed the first medical marijuana initiative in 1996.

Use or abuse?

You might not like a recreational drug that your brother takes or that he drinks a six pack a day. But that's not your life or your call once you have applied the test often used to determine addiction: Is it interfering with the other aspects of a person's life?

If the answer is no, you should probably let it go. It's tough to convince somebody to stop doing something that brings pleasure. Just ask any little boy who's promised to stop when he needs glasses.

IS INPATIENT REHAB NECESSARY?

The answer to that one is a big fat maybe.

We no longer believe that people with substance abuse issues must bottom out before it is possible to rehabilitate them. We have also learned that some people can be highly functional despite major addictions.

That doesn't mean that they might not need help in ending destructive addictive patterns and behaviors.

We hear most often about celebrities going to rehab, often under messy circumstances that all but require an enforced absence from polite society. But regular folks can and do benefit from facing addiction in a controlled setting, and for some people that's the only thing that works.

This kind of help does not come cheap. The Affordable Care Act now requires insurance parity for medical and mental health/substance abuse services, but the details of implementation are still being, well, tweaked.

POST-TRAUMATIC STRESS DISORDER

We first started hearing about PTSD (post-traumatic stress disorder) in relation to Vietnam veterans suffering from a war-related condition that had previously been known as shell shock, battle fatigue, soldier's heart, or the thousand-yard stare.

Perhaps because previous generations had been forced to ignore this sign of perceived weakness, it took baby boomers who didn't mind making a fuss to bring it to the attention of a broader public.

Today the term PTSD is used to describe the aftermath of dozens of different types of events, from auto accidents to muggings to ... well, pretty much anything. This expansion of nomenclature isn't as helpful as it might be, though anything which allows people with problems to seek help is probably a good thing.

For the record, there is no time limit on PTSD. It can kick in ten minutes after an event, or forty years down the road.

And keeping it bottled up inside is not necessarily a useful strategy.

If you are dealing with a military veteran and you think this may be an issue that should be addressed, check with local veterans' organizations or the VA for guidance.

THE ANONYMOUS COMMUNITY

The greatest resource available to people facing substance abuse problems in contemporary America remains the Anonymous community.

Twelve Step programs now include 200 specialized areas of addictive behaviors. Confidentiality and anonymity are the central tenets of them all.

Alcoholics Anonymous officially began in 1938, with Narcotics Anonymous breaking off in 1953 to address specific issues of drug addiction. Nobody knows how many people have been positively affected by these programs over the past three-quarters of a century, but if you include the families and friends of participants, we have to be talking millions. If you haven't spent your entire life in a cave, you undoubtedly know some of these people.

In addition to programs and help for those facing addiction firsthand, related programs such as Al-Anon, Alateen and Adult Children of Alcoholics help family members deal with the secondary problems and repercussions of substance abuse. If you are dealing with somebody whose behaviors concern you, starting with one of these support groups can be just the ticket.

Twelve Step-related meetings are everywhere—on land, at sea, and in cyberspace.

These groups pride themselves on accessibility and the default meeting place for many has traditionally been church basements. Many local organizations offer 24-hour hotlines because, face it, people don't always come to the decision that they need addiction help during regular business hours. To get information on specific meeting locations, you need to deal directly with the local organization. That's to protect everybody's privacy, and you'll appreciate the level of protection should you or your sibling become active in the Anonymous community.

All Twelve Step programs are by definition anonymous and respect for that anonymity is taken very seriously.

ADDITIONAL INFORMATION

Mental Health

American Association for Geriatric Psychiatry
www.aagponline.org/

American Psychological Association
www.apa.org/

Anxiety and Depression Association of America
www.adaa.org

Brain & Behavior Research Foundation
www.bbrfoundation.org

Depressed Test: Am I Depressed?
www.depressedtest.com/

Depression and Bipolar Support Alliance
www.dbsalliance.org
800.826.3632

D for Depression & Depressive Psychological Disorders
www.depressiond.com/

Mental Health America
www.mentalhealthamerica.net/
800.969.6642

NAMI: National Alliance on Mental Illness
www.nami.org/
800.950.6264

International OCD Foundation: Obsessive-Compulsive Disorder
www.ocfoundation.org

SARDAA: Schizophrenia and Related Disorders Alliance of America
www.sardaa.org/

Schizophrenia.com: In-Depth Schizophrenia Information and Support
www.schizophrenia.com/

Schizophrenia Research Forum
www.schizophreniaforum.org/

Substance Abuse and Mental Health Services Administration
www.samhsa.gov/
800.662.HELP

• • • • •

Ava T. Albrecht and Charles Herrick
100 Questions & Answers About Depression
Jones and Bartlett, 2011

Carol Berman
100 Questions & Answers About Panic Disorder
Jones and Bartlett, 2010

Jay Carter and Bobbi Dempsey
The Complete Idiot's Guide to Bipolar Disorder
Idiot Guides, 2009

Katie d'Ath and Rob Wilson
Managing OCD with CBT for Dummies
For Dummies, 2016

Lynn E. DeLisi
100 Questions & Answers About Schizophrenia: Painful Minds
Jones and Bartlett, 2011

Troy DuFrene and Bryce M. Hyman
Coping with OCD: Practical Strategies for Living Well with Obsessive-Compulsive Disorder
New Harbinger Publications, 2008

Candida Fink and Joe Kraynak
Bipolar Disorder for Dummies, 2nd Edition
For Dummies, 2012

Richard Day Gore and Juliann Garey
Voices of Bipolar Disorder: The Healing Companion: Stories for Courage, Comfort and Strength
La Chance Publishing, 2010

Bryce Hyman and Cherlene Pedrick
The OCD Workbook: Your Guide to Breaking Free from Obsessive-Compulsive Disorder
New Harbinger Publications, 2010

Jerome Levine and Irene S. Levine
Schizophrenia for Dummies
For Dummies, 2008

David J. Miklowitz
The Bipolar Disorder Survival Guide, 2nd Edition
Guilford Press, 2010

Mark D. Miller and Charles F. Reynolds III
Depression and Anxiety in Later Life: What Everyone Needs to Know
Johns Hopkins Press, 2012

National Institute of Mental Health
Understanding Schizophrenia: Signs and Symptoms
Amazon Kindle, 2012

National Institute of Mental Health, National Institutes of Health, and US Department of Health and Human Services
Schizophrenia: Causes, Symptoms, Signs, Diagnosis and Treatments, Revised
CreateSpace, 2012

Susan J. Noonan
Managing Your Depression: What You Can Do to Feel Better
Johns Hopkins Press, 2013

Amy L. Sutton, ed.
Depression Sourcebook, 3rd Edition
Omnigraphics Health Reference Series Health Reference Series, 2012

Substance Abuse

Adult Children of Alcoholics
www.adultchildren.org/

Al-Anon Family Groups
www.al-anon.org/
888.4AL.ANON

Alcoholics Anonymous
www.aa.org

Narcotics Anonymous
www.na.org
818.773.9999 x771

Subject Abuse and Mental Health Services Administration
www.samhsa.gov/
800.662.HELP

WHEN YOU ARE THE PATIENT

Of all the people involved in a SibCare situation, the one who is both most important and least interested in being involved is usually the patient.

When you are the patient, you are immersed in all kinds of things that you never thought you'd have to face. You want nothing to do with any of it, but you often need to make serious decisions Right This Second. Scary words are being tossed around, everything you've scheduled is going right out the window, and you have totally lost control of your life.

This is not the time to be Superman or Wonder Woman. Accept the loss of control and do your best to be gracious about it, even if it requires banging your fist through the wall. This is a time to marshal your resources, consult with family and friends whose wisdom and opinions you trust, obtain as much medical information as you can stand without having your head explode, and then get into bed with the covers over your head.

It all sucks, big time. It's not fair.

Aunt Elspeth never had a kind word for anybody, and she lived to be 104. Uncle Jed drinks like an Irish innkeeper, smokes three packs a day, eats nothing but saturated fats, and just turned 87. Whereas you, who exercised regularly and ate properly and did everything right—at least most of the time—are now facing life-threatening illness.

Your personality is not going to change. Neither is anybody else's. You need to work with who you are and what you know about each other—your siblings, your friends, and your family—and how you interrelate.

Everybody is likely to be in some kind of denial, and yours may be at the top of the pyramid. It takes time to process unwelcome medical information, and more time to figure out treatment options, finances, and the mechanics of implementation. However, time may be a central issue, particularly if your situation was precipitated by a particular event that needs immediate attention.

ADVOCACY

You need an advocate.

Even the most self-reliant person is at a huge disadvantage when dealing with medical issues while simultaneously experiencing pain, drug disorientation, emotional upheaval, stress of all varieties, and the unanswerable question of *Why me?*

If you are able, figure out who in your immediate circle is best suited to advocacy and put that person to work. Make it clear who's handling things and others will gratefully recede into the woodwork and take up other jobs. If somebody's feelings are going to be hurt by your choice, try to think of something else that person can do and pitch it as important. (Or have your advocate think of something else and pitch it to Miss Ever-So-Sensitive; that's part of what the advocate is for.)

Your advocate should be with you at medical appointments and consultations, armed with a notepad and predetermined questions. Lots of us experience white coat amnesia in stressful situations, forgetting what we wanted to know and ask about until that moment in the parking lot later when it all comes flooding back. We may also get distracted and let important information slip right past.

Write things down.

Your advocate can ask the tough questions, particularly if your denial level is still high, but everything will be a lot easier if you can share in advance what your primary concerns are. Some examples:

- Difficult treatments and potential side-effects?
- Therapy problems?
- Paying for it all?
- Making decisions about how to handle this unfortunate hand you've just been dealt?

- Understanding what cards are in that hand?
- Short-term prognosis?
- Long-term prognosis?
- Whether there will even *be* a long term?

The best person for this role may not be the most obvious. If your spouse is dazed and dithering, you may want to ask your toughest, most capable child to become your advocate. Or the friend who got the school board to back down on a major local issue. Or your tough-ass sister-in-law, or your brother whose persistence has always annoyed everybody. Traits which are normally difficult to deal with can suddenly become incredibly useful. Don't let your assumptions and prejudices keep you from getting the right help for the right job.

You and your advocate will both benefit from reading Jessie Gruman's *AfterShock: What to Do When the Doctor Gives You—or Someone you Love—a Devastating Diagnosis.* It's filled with practical material presented in a caring tone. And it will bring up things you never thought of.

Advocacy is discussed at greater length in the "Information Gathering and Advocacy" chapter.

DETERMINING THE FACTS

Somebody needs to be learning about your medical problem in at least enough detail to understand both the nature of the beast and how it is battled. That person doesn't need to be you and it doesn't even need to be somebody who will make decisions on these issues. You're looking for a person who's comfortable with research and the internet, or who at least knows how to order copies of the books suggested as additional resources on particular subjects throughout this volume.

You may decide you want to know only the basics, or you may choose to immerse yourself in the chemistry footnotes in journal reports of potential treatments. Your call, so long as *somebody* is looking at the details if you're not able to. Keeping facts straight matters in these kinds of situations, and is covered in greater detail in the chapter on "Learning What You Need to

Know."

GRACIOUSLY ACCEPTING HELP

Let people help you. For many of us, that is the hardest thing of all.

You may feel you are just fine with the medical situation and totally on top of it all. You thoroughly understand the ramifications of your treatment, have ordered your post-chemo wig, and just finished packaging and freezing three months' worth of food for the dinners you won't be cooking. Or maybe you've told your coworkers you'll be back two weeks after surgery and assured your son and daughter-in-law that there's no reason whatsoever to postpone that trip to Europe.

Here's the thing. You may think you'll snap right back, and maybe you will. But sometimes it takes longer than you expect to recover from surgery, radiation, chemotherapy, rehab, or whatever else gets flung onto your medical plate. This is not cause for embarrassment or shame. It's just a fact of life.

Furthermore, you need to be gentle enough on yourself to allow that extra time. You may be a captain of industry with hundreds of people waiting on your decisions, but you know what? If your plane went down, those decisions would still somehow get made, though perhaps not as well as you'd do it.

Of course you are important, and what you do is significant. But it isn't the only thing going on right now, and if you are the only one in the room who refuses to recognize that, you just make things tougher on everybody.

SELF-PITY

A certain amount of self-pity is not only a good thing, but probably essential.

Dammit, this was *not* what you had in mind! You had *plans.* You have every reason and right to feel sorry for yourself. But after an initial period of bereft withdrawal, you do need to get up and get back into this new game you have suddenly begun playing.

Keep in mind that martyrdom is not an attractive quality.

This doesn't mean you aren't entitled to cry and scream and wail. In fact, you probably should. But if you make complaint your primary form of communication, the folks who want to help you will feel less inclined to do so.

You don't need to be Little Merry Sunshine all the time, but if you answer every query of "How are you doing?" with an exhaustive symptom recital or by bursting into tears, you'll find the question asked a lot less frequently.

There will also be fewer folks around to do the asking.

MATTERS OF FAITH AND RELIGION

If you are a member of a faith community, this is an excellent time to get those people involved. Your faith can be a real comfort as you face an uncertain future, and the folks who share your beliefs will have a pretty good idea how to keep that comfort coming. They also have a tendency to be good people who genuinely want to help. You should let them, whether it's driving you to appointments, or dropping off casseroles, or just calling to see how you're doing.

You may, however, find that people with different beliefs from yours will want you to get you on their own religious bandwagon. *You are under no obligation to climb aboard.* Thank them politely for their concern, tell them that you are not interested in having that discussion, and feel no need to agree to anything.

This one can get tricky. If somebody who cares about you is certain you are headed straight for hell unless you don't change your belief structure right this minute, that person may be highly motivated to save your soul. That person may, in fact, become a royal pain in the butt.

On the other hand, it can't possibly hurt to have folks of different beliefs praying to their respective deities in their customary fashions, even if the custom has nothing to do with what you normally believe. If somebody says he's praying for you, just say thank you and smile.

PRIVACY MEANS MORE
THAN A HIPAA FORM

Build in some barriers. It may be your illness, but you don't have to be the social secretary, too.

If you don't want to see people, you don't have to. You don't need to stagger out of bed to answer the doorbell, or pick up phone calls from well-meaning people who want to know how they can help when you haven't got a clue. It's perfectly all right to ignore knocks on the door that you aren't expecting and to screen your calls. Likewise, you can and should delete emails from irritating people or folks sending prayer chains of kneeling puppies to a lifelong atheist. Delete, delete, delete. You can build up a nice rhythm, and it feels good, too.

If you can install some form of gatekeeping assistance, do so.

Have somebody else answer the door or put a note by the bell saying PLEASE DO NOT DISTURB. Send calls on your cell phone straight to message, and do the same for any other answering machine or voicemail system. Most phones will let you block particular callers, too, sending them right to message.

If you don't want to talk to *anybody*, let people know you'd prefer to communicate by email, or say (preferably through your gatekeeper) that you'll call them back soon. And if you don't call them back soon—or ever—*do not* feel guilty about it.

Do whatever is comfortable for you and don't feel obligated to respond to everybody. You're sick, after all, so the Excuse-o-Meter is always going to swing favorably in your direction.

The trick here is to realize that the barriers shouldn't be high enough to keep out the folks you really *do* need and want to see. So tell your gatekeeper that you only want to see Jan and Bob and your minister, and let the gatekeeper do the dirty work of turning others away. When you're ready to widen the circle, the gatekeeper can let those people know.

INFORMATION SHARING

How much to share with others may or may not be up to you.

If you were in a coma for three weeks after an automobile accident, a lot of notifications and decisions have already taken place and there's nothing you can do about it. Other people probably know a lot more about what's been happening than you do, and they'll be bringing *you* up to date.

But if you got a surprise diagnosis after a routine physical or when you made a fast appointment for something you figured was pretty minor, you've got more leeway.

You can take some time to process the information and decide what to do next, and if you're retired it's even easier to quietly slip away for a spell. Tell people you have the flu if they're persistent, but don't lie to your immediate family or other close friends and relatives. At least not for long. These are the people you are going to need to rely upon through whatever is coming next.

Swear people to secrecy if you wish, and if you know somebody is a blabbermouth, discuss how to control her with others in your circle. Just don't try to carry too much alone. Not only does that place too heavy a burden on you, it also robs the people who care about you of an opportunity to show their love. In ways that matter, when it matters.

I am continually amazed at how many people who live in a very public eye are able to keep physical problems private, sometimes until the very moment of a death announcement. They tend to already have built-in barriers, of course, in the form of staff, assistants, money, and figurative drawbridges to be pulled up at multiple residences.

And yet sometimes the ones who manage to get away with it are people who are extraordinarily social. I was stunned to hear that Nora Ephron had died, for instance—but even more stunned when I realized that this most sociable and open of women had also managed to hide an illness of many years' duration from just about all of her friends as well.

PAPERWORK

Get your paperwork in order.

I know, I know. This really isn't all that serious and you don't intend to die just now, thank you very much. Besides, everybody knows what you want, and it's bad luck to think about it and you don't have all that much stuff anyway.

Guess what? Everybody *doesn't* know what you want, and even those close to you may have different ideas on the subject. People get into horrible fights over medical decisions and sometimes even wind up in court when their relatives are not clear about preferred care.

So let's look at this as a Purely Hypothetical Situation.

If, God forbid, something unfortunate should happen while you're in the hospital, who will decide how you should be treated? Your children? Your ex-wife? Your sister-in-law? That doctor whose name you can't even remember? Some judge whose primary qualification for appointed office was nepotism?

The "Legal Paperwork" chapter will walk you through what you need to do and why. Do it. You do not need a lawyer, though if this is the way you normally and comfortably handle business, it's an easy default.

The single most important thing you need is Advance Directives. This will designate who can make medical decisions for you and clarify what type of treatment you prefer in the Purely Hypothetical Situation where something unforeseen has happened. Make sure your paperwork is properly signed and witnessed. In some instances, paperwork should be notarized.

Be sure that your advocate and/or other appropriate parties are aware of your wishes and have copies of everything.

Your doctor's office and any hospital where you are having procedures done as an outpatient or an inpatient should also have copies. Get them scanned into your file as soon as they exist.

THE BALANCING ACT
OF CONTROL

You may find yourself debilitated, disoriented, distracted, and exhausted.

Even if this is your normal state, you're probably the one most aware of how much everything has changed, and how quickly. You can bluff to some degree, but unless you live in a bell jar, others are likely to recognize that all is not exactly hunky dory at the moment.

If people know you're not well, they may treat you differently. It's hard not to, really. If you think about your own past behavior, you'll probably be able to verify this pretty quickly, with a smidgen of shame and embarrassment.

But you also have some control over the way people act in your presence. If you don't want people to be all weepy and gloomy around you, by all means tell them to cheer up or take a hike.

Indeed, it's a good idea to steer clear of doomsayers as a matter of principle, particularly if you tend to be one yourself. This kind of thing can move into a downward spiral of self-pity and despair all too quickly. Do you know somebody who routinely starts sentences with: "I don't want to worry you, but…"? Well, let me tell you two things. One, that person *does* want to worry you, and two, it probably isn't going to be helpful or friendly advice anyway.

Practice saying, "I don't want to talk about that" until you can do it with a straight face and repeat it until the person shuts up. Also practice saying, "Could you just shut up?" so you'll have some backup if quiet civility doesn't work.

Keep a sense of humor.

ADDITIONAL INFORMATION

Jessie Gruman
AfterShock: What to do When the Doctor Gives You—or Someone You Love—a Devastating Diagnosis
Walker & Co., 2007

SECTION NINE:

END OF LIFE ISSUES

When Hank Williams sang that he'd never get out of this world alive, he probably didn't realize that he himself would never hit thirty.

The reality is that nobody gets a pass on death.

The privileged may have a better shot at getting state-of-the-art care and treatment. Still, if sufficient means and the will to live were the only requirements, George Harrison would be strumming his guitar on his beach in Maui, Steve Jobs would be inventing things that nobody ever thought of before, and Gilda Radner would have her own comedy network.

THE FIVE STAGES

We are all familiar with the five stages of grief first identified and named by Elisabeth Kubler-Ross: Denial, Anger, Bargaining, Depression, and Acceptance.

What we don't always realize is that these can come and go, don't necessarily appear in order, and often apply with equal logic to severe or chronic illness.

It can be useful to recognize that you are going through these stages, whether during the early part of an illness or its final stages, though little purpose is served in dwelling too long on any of it. Does it really matter whether you are grappling with denial or anger, when you need to get your sister to her fourth medical appointment of the week?

When I was younger and more naïve, not long after my brother's brain tumor diagnosis in 1994, I remember having dinner with a childhood friend who was now a practicing physician. "Oh, I worked through those stages already," I told him.

His reply shook me, and turned out to be right on target: "You may find yourself going through them all again, maybe more than once."

In practical terms of care for a sibling who is doing poorly, you may find these five stages a useful gauge of where other siblings or loved ones are on the continuum. That awareness may allow you to work more easily with them—and to get them to work with you—as you all head down this rough and lonely road.

A RISING SENSE OF LOSS

No matter how prepared you may think you are to lose a sibling, you can never be entirely ready. As you move through end-of-life activities and motions, it is common and normal to experience a wrenching sense of impending loss. This can't be happening, your heart tells you, even as your mind is weighing options, making phone calls, coordinating care, and doing your utmost to hold things together for everybody.

You can ignore this sense of loss, and a lot of the time you don't have much choice because there is so much to do. But don't be afraid to give in to it now and then. Tears are cathartic, screaming in your car provides excellent release, and if you are willing and able to share your feelings with other relatives, you will probably find them mirrored.

I wouldn't be so silly as to claim that a sorrow shared is a sorrow halved, but it *is* a sorrow shared. Do it.

PAPERWORK AND FINANCES

Now is when some of the most important paperwork of all comes into play.

People hate to think they are going to die and many believe that if they put it on paper it will happen and if they don't, it won't. Or, conversely, they try to bring the subject up with their children, who pooh-pooh the topic: "Don't be silly,

Mom. You're going to be around when [insert event which is well down the road, such as a one-year-old's wedding]. Don't talk that way!"

The end result is too often an unconscious patient in ICU while the kids argue about what to do next and what Dad really meant that time when he got so loaded and said such-and-such. Some of these cases end up in court at a time when everybody ought to be uniting in familial care for a loved one who is severely ill and may be dying.

End-of-life paperwork needs to be in every medical file and hospital chart and on the refrigerator door if the patient is at home. If there is a DNR (do not resuscitate) or POLST order with preferred treatment options in place, it needs to be in the hands of paramedics, ER staff, and assisted living or nursing home personnel. You can find this all in the chapter on "Legal Paperwork."

It is far better to be repetitive with this information than to run the risk of some medical action taking place that is contrary to the patient's wishes. If the patient isn't conscious, that information-sharing falls to the caregiving team.

You can put all of these documents in PDF form into an app or folder on your smartphone, which will make them accessible to anybody who needs to see something *right now* and will allow you to email them instantly to anybody who needs them.

CONTRADICTIONS

People visualize themselves dying at home surrounded by loved ones, with some favorite music playing softly and a breeze coming through the open springtime window. That's the way everybody used to do it (unless they were in battle), and we all know of similar instances in the very recent past.

The reality, however, is that people are more likely to be hooked up to all kinds of equipment and monitors and machines in the Intensive Care Unit where family can visit for five minutes an hour.

Quality of life and death are concepts that people don't

talk about much, though there is always a flurry of discussion after some deaths, statements that range from "I don't ever want to go through anything like that" to "I can't believe she gave up so easily."

Most folks are pretty much decided about their end-of-life desires, whether articulated or not. They mostly want to die peacefully at home with loved ones, and Medicare data show that about a third of patients over 65 do die that way. However, more than half die in hospitals or nursing homes.

In addition to being a cold clinical setting, hospital death is expensive. One health care analysis showed that 17% of the Medicare budget was spent on the last six months of patients' lives. Medicare estimates that a quarter of its spending is applied to the five percent of participants who die each year, an average of over $20,000 per Medicare hospital death.

WHO'S INVOLVED IN FINAL DECISIONS?

While it may have been difficult to get relatives and friends to pitch in for such mundane caregiving chores as transportation and meal preparation, folks tend to pop up with their unsolicited ideas and opinions in the latter stages of an illness. Folks who were conspicuous by their absence are suddenly very much present and eager to tell everybody what to do.

Try to view this as a challenge born out of love and concern, even when your strongest instinct is a desire to deck the latecomer. But if decisions have already been made and are in effect, make it equally clear to dissidents that you need support rather than interference.

If your sibling has her end-of-life paperwork in order, all of this will be considerably easier. Make sure that those formalized wishes are available to everyone who may need them.

RELIGIOUS MATTERS

When people begin to consider end-of-life options and possibilities, many lean more heavily on their religious beliefs and faith communities. Overall, this is usually a good thing, since faith helps bring people through difficult experiences and a relationship with a greater power can be a huge comfort in a time of impending loss.

In addition, faith communities can provide tremendous support and assistance through this very rough period, for both spiritual and practical matters.

The ideal circumstance is one where everybody involved is in general agreement on religious matters, sharing the same belief system and maybe even the same physical church. Usually, however, you can't count on that kind of unanimity. Things may therefore get a little tricky.

Keep in mind that the single most important player here is the person at its center. Her beliefs are the ones that should matter the most and take priority. And those may be anywhere along a continuum from atheism at one end to devout practice of a specific religion at the other.

The wartime adage that there are no atheists in foxholes often comes into play as well. Some people approaching the end of their lives find that while atheism or agnosticism was quite comfortable in earlier years, they are now inclined to hedge their bets a bit. This may mean a return to the religion of childhood or turning to an entirely new faith system.

No matter what you personally may believe, you don't have any business forcing your faith on your sibling. This is true even if your religion specifically exhorts you to do so, and if you believe that your sister will suffer mightily in the afterlife without your guidance.

Generally when people feel this strongly about religious differences, the subject has come up before. If that's the case, it may be easier to accept that your sister's decisions on these matters are hers alone. Not yours, not her husband's, not her children's, not her friends'.

Nor should you keep harping on it. Quoting scripture endlessly or praying over somebody who doesn't want you to is really poor manners and achieves nothing but resentment.

Similarly, once your sister has made her feelings known, you don't have any business bringing your own priest or minister or rabbi or guru into her life unless you have her express permission to do so.

However.

There's nothing to prevent you from praying on your own, or from soliciting prayers and good thoughts from anyone you know or encounter. These may be highly formalized or very casual, and they may be in direct conflict with what you personally believe. That doesn't matter. What matters is that somebody cares.

My own feeling is that in bad situations it can't possibly hurt to have concerned people praying to any deities available to listen.

Try to keep in mind that people have their own ways of dealing with adversity and that *everybody* is having a hard time with all of this. Don't get angry if you can possibly avoid it. Enough wars have been fought over religion already. Your family doesn't have to tack on another one, especially at a time when you ought to be supporting one another.

Respect your sibling's beliefs, practice your own, and let others use their own faith systems for strength and comfort.

WHEN THE SCENE
BEGINS TO SHIFT

Some illnesses arrive bearing their own finality and others drift in that direction over months and years. In the case of major illness, matters often take on a life of their own. Once everyone has been swept into the stream of care and treatment and concern it may be difficult to step back and realistically assess the larger picture.

Sometimes it is the patient who decides that it is time to stop fighting. Sometimes the patient is the only one who's still willing to fight. Every situation is different and you need to look at it in terms of your own family specifics and try to work together accordingly.

In many terminal illnesses, a time comes when you realize you're playing a zero-sum game. Treatment is no longer likely to make a significant difference.

Quality of life becomes the issue, and it's interesting to note that physicians who are more familiar with the mechanics and pathways of death seem to understand that quite clearly, particularly for themselves. They recognize that just because a treatment is available, that doesn't mean it's worth pursuing.

If three months of hideous treatment will prolong life by three months, what exactly has been gained? Is it worth it financially or emotionally? Is it worth fighting about? And who's doing that fighting, anyway? The patient or those who will be left behind?

This is also the time when folks start to look for last ditch solutions. Surely there's some experimental treatment, clinical trial, new doctor, herbal concoction, or miracle that will fix everything. This often carries an air of desperation, particularly when people have been previously unable or unwilling to confront medical realities.

The patient's loved ones may find themselves in sharp disagreement. One person or faction wants to fight on, while another wants to look into palliative care and hospice. Ugliness can erupt here, particularly if some Johnny-come-lately is insisting that there has to be something else that can be done.

As matters swirl around these decisions, try not to make promises to your sibling that you may not be able to keep. This just sets you up to feel guilty later.

It may seem easier to agree to something with your fingers crossed than to explain why it won't work, but compromise if you can. "I'll do my best" covers a lot of territory without promising to deliver something beyond your control.

If your family is on different pages here, or maybe not even in the same book, keep your arguments away from the patient unless you are absolutely certain that the patient is willing to express and stand up for a previously articulated position.

Above all, remember that hearing often can and does remain functional even when somebody is unconscious or comatose. Don't say *anything* in the vicinity of the patient that you don't want the patient to hear. Period.

THE MYTH OF DEATH PANELS

In recent years as health care has undergone major national re-evaluation and reform, we have heard intermittently about so-called Death Panels, which do not currently exist in any form in the United States.

This discussion began during the debate over passage of the Affordable Care Act, which originally included a provision that would have reimbursed doctors for a one-time discussion of end-of-life options with patients. This type of candid and matter-of-fact discussion happens all too rarely right now, though it would help simplify and clarify many issues. That ACA provision was dropped in the resultant brouhaha when a politician characterized these physician-patient discussions as death panels.

Medicare is currently moving to make end-of-life discussions a regular part of the medical process.

SAYING GOODBYE

If family members are far-flung, matters can get complicated. Are there friends and relatives who will want to come and say goodbye? Does your sister want to see or talk to them? This is a highly individual matter.

Some people make a particular effort to say goodbye to people who have been important to them, while others want only to be left alone. If somebody feels terrible and looks like hell, she may not be inclined to receive, and you need to listen to her. You might suggest that she can speak briefly with people on the phone as a compromise.

Respect the patient's wishes as much as you can, but try not to be too rigid. If there's somebody in your sister's life who's been long estranged and you know that person would like to mend the relationship, tell your sister and ask for guidance. If she says no, respect that, though depending on circumstances you might also suggest that person send a card or letter which could help smooth matters and avoid regrets.

In far-flung families, there are logistical considerations as well. When to come? Where to stay? How long to stay? Expense can be a very real issue, along with other work and family responsibilities. If somebody can only afford to make one trip, I personally would always vote for showing up to say goodbye rather than attending a funeral or memorial service.

Try not to confuse wishes with realities. But if you're trying to heal old wounds, or to assemble folks from far away, don't wait too long.

WHAT, WHERE, AND HOW MUCH?

End-of-life care may take place in the patient's home, in a hospital, in a nursing home or skilled nursing facility, or in a dedicated hospice facility. If the patient is conscious and able to participate in decision-making, include him wherever possible. Beyond that, this is not a democratic process. The primary family caregivers should make these decisions based on their understanding of the patient's written and previously expressed wishes, as well as the convenience of those same caregivers.

PALLIATIVE CARE

In recent years we've heard much more about palliative care, which is generally a component of end-of-life care, though by no means limited to the dying. It is not uncommon for someone with a chronic, non-terminal condition to have palliative care as well as treatments aimed at the illness itself.

Palliative care is medical treatment designed to relieve pain, symptoms, and stress caused by serious illnesses. Its goal is not to cure the disease, but to improve the patient's quality of life. The objective here is comfort, to the greatest degree possible.

HOSPICE

Hospice in many ways represents a return to the ways of yesteryear, when a person who was dying did so at home in his own bed, cared for in his final days and hours by loved ones.

The definition is a little broader now, and hospice care may also occur in a skilled nursing or dedicated hospice facility. Forty-four percent of Medicare beneficiaries who died in 2010 used hospice, up dramatically from 23 percent only ten years earlier.

Hospice care is a team effort, and a hospice team customarily includes the patient, family caregivers, doctors, nurses, home health aides, clergy, and social workers.

Not everybody will be there all the time, of course, but team members coordinate care to assure that what is needed is available. Special equipment is often brought in, including hospital beds. Your area may offer a choice of hospice providers, and if that's the case it's worth talking to people who are familiar with their differences to find the right situation for your family.

Palliative care is central to hospice, though treatment aimed at cure or remission is generally discontinued. The goal is to make the patient comfortable and to allow family members to be present without bearing responsibility for medical matters.

Medicare, Medicaid, and most private insurance covers hospice, a win-win situation that generally costs a lot less and provides a lot more. Indeed, Medicare covered 84% of the patients in hospice in 2011. To participate in hospice with Medicare, the patient must be willing to stop any treatments aimed at a cure, though medications unrelated to the terminal illness will still be covered. Federally funded hospice care requires a doctor's certification that a patient is terminal, with less than six months to live. This doesn't mean that a patient will be kicked out at six months and a day, though a new six-month certification will be required.

Copious information about hospice is available

through several national organizations, and the Hospice Association of America even offers a "Hospice Patient's Bill of Rights."

If you have any doubts at all about hospice care, take a look at the number of obituaries which specifically ask for donations to hospice programs in lieu of flowers.

ENDING LIFE SUPPORT

Who gets to decide when to discontinue life support in situations where it's already in place can often become a legal issue. Medical facilities don't like to do this and if someone has been inadvertently placed on life support (which can happen when an unconscious patient arrives in the emergency room) matters become complicated.

In this case there will inevitably be Official Procedures and you will have to deal with them. Literally pulling the plug yourself is not an option, even if you know that's what your brother would want. You'll end up in jail and he may or may not be physically considered alive after the attempt.

This is perhaps the single best reason for having Advance Directives in place.

PHYSICIAN-ASSISTED SUICIDE

Physician-assisted suicide is currently legal in five states: California, Oregon, Vermont and Washington by legislation, and Montana by court ruling. All require residency. It is illegal in the other 45 states and the District of Columbia.

The national movement to approve assisted suicide was begun by Derek Humphry who founded the Hemlock Society in 1980 and named it for the poison taken by Socrates. That organization later morphed and merged with others, resulting in the formation of the more neutrally-named Compassion & Choices in 2005.

The decidedly creepy Dr. Jack Kevorkian, AKA Dr. Death, brought public attention to the issue in the 1990s by actively involving himself in a hundred assisted deaths. He was convicted of second degree murder (after three previous acquittals and a mistrial in other cases) and served eight years in Michigan before being paroled on the condition that he no longer assist in deaths or provide care to anyone over 62 or disabled. He himself has since died.

This is an extremely sensitive topic and anyone who wants more information can find it through either Compassion & Choices or Final Exit, the two organizations which are primarily involved with these issues.

THE ARRANGEMENTS
NOBODY WANT TO MAKE

The funerals of yesteryear were very pro forma, with somber traditional hymns followed by a procession to the cemetery and coffee back at somebody's house. As a teenager, I was once sent to buy an assortment of cigarettes for just such a funeral. Yes, really.

Today you are as likely to find a Celebration of Life held a couple of months later, with shared reminiscences and a joyous party afterward. Note: You can celebrate and cry at the same time. I've done that, too.

In some instances, a Celebration of Life may take place while the central figure is actually still alive. This had never occurred to me until a recent gathering from far-flung corners of the country was held for a friend on the downslope of a very bad diagnosis.

What your family prefers may be set by religious tradition or be wide open for discussion—and sometimes survivors can get into major arguments about what to do and who should do it. It is not uncommon for the terminally ill to aid in planning their own services or even write their own obituaries. Conversely, sometimes the dying person is adamant about wanting no service at all. Or about where and when and how ashes should be scattered.

Dying people can get bossy.

Unless religious requirements dictate otherwise, you have a bit of time leeway in making these decisions, even if you wait to do everything until after the fact. Some of the nicest memorial services I've attended occurred after the passage of time, and some of the most rewarding have been the simplest.

If money is an issue, don't let yourself be guilt-tripped into spending more than necessary. On anything. It is not unseemly to comparison shop.

If there are people who don't even realize that your brother has been sick, you might want to start making "serious illness" contact with people around the time he goes into hospice. This will save you having to tell the whole story again and again later, when it will be even more painful. You may also find yourself making some nice reconnections with people who've been important in various ways in your sibling's life, and quite possibly also your own.

You can use the same care networks and telephone contacts you've had in place all along to let local people know: church, neighbors, co-workers. And if you have a chance, you can try to track down folks who are *really* out of contact, the ones you maybe should have looked for a year ago when all this began.

Social networking can be useful and efficient, though I find it jarring to learn of a friend's death on Facebook, and probably always will. Traditional newspaper obituaries are particularly helpful for spreading the word in a hurry if a service is planned soon. These are now sold by the column inch in many places, with an additional photo fee. That photo doesn't have to be recent, however. If a picture from thirty years ago sums up exactly what your sister was like, go ahead and use it.

DEATH OF A SIBLING

The loss of a sibling gets short shrift in our society.

A mother or father, a child, a spouse—these are all recognized as monumental losses, altering your life in expected and familiar ways. Commonplace, almost, as one ages. But society has no standard expectations where sibling loss is concerned.

"They say that when you lose a sibling, you lose your

childhood," a friend whose brother and only sib died of cancer told me.

To a strong and haunting degree, I believe she is right. Your siblings remember you when you were little, before your first bra or the embarrassment of your changing voice. They recall the sour fruit on the backyard cherry tree and learning to swim at the lake in the summer and the goofy mutt who kept running away. They shared your room, for better or worse, and their classroom performance affected what teachers later expected from you or vice versa. They pitched balls you swung at in the summer street, including the one you hit right through a neighbor's window.

I had been living in the SibCare world for years, but I never made major connections about my own family's significant sibling losses until I read *The Empty Room* by Elizabeth DeVita-Raeburn.

My father lost two of his three brothers before he was fifty, including one who died accidentally as a teen during World War II when all three of the older boys were off in the military. When my mother died suddenly at fifty, I honestly wondered whether her only sibling, a sister in Ohio, would even come to the funeral. Their relations had been badly strained by the issue of care for their father, who had lived with us and was an unwitting but constant source of friction. (My aunt did come, of course.)

The magnitude of loss is even stronger among one set of my cousins, who began as a foursome: two boys and two girls. They lost their father as young teens, then the older sister when she was 21. Both were suicides. The younger brother drowned at 53, leaving just the older brother and younger sister, both of whom took exceptionally good care of themselves.

But you never know. Two weeks before my brother's relatively expected death, my hale and hearty male cousin had a massive heart attack at 63 while reading in front of a freshly built fire with his beloved dog at his feet.

And then there was one.

What little information exists on sibling loss tends to

focus more on childhood death, which DeVita-Raeburn believes has been historically minimized because higher infant and childhood mortality rates in the past made it seem more common, somehow normal. She also suggests that family roles are sometimes reassigned (think Kennedys) in a concept known as "living for two."

Childhood death is regarded primarily as a parental loss, wherein kids are expected to care for their parents and each other—suppressing grief, and Being Good. If the lost sibling was difficult or had been very ill, children may feel a sense of relief that they recognize as inappropriate and feel even more guilty about.

As for what happens when adult siblings die, we're making that one up as we go along.

GRIEF

Grief knows no boundaries. Grief has no rules. It is as universal as life itself and as unique as DNA.

It can be predictable, of course, appearing at designated times and places. It's expected that you'll grieve when delivered a definitive and deadly diagnosis. When the last possible treatment fails. When the light goes dimmer in the one you love. When that light flickers for the final time and then is extinguished forever.

Everyone knows and anticipates that you will grieve in the first hours and days and weeks when a loved one dies. Our society recognizes and respects that. But there is also a get-on-with-business attitude that slips into place shortly thereafter, when acquaintances say, "I'm sorry for your loss" and then expect you to leap right back into whatever you were doing when the earth's axis changed forever.

Grief can also slither into the most unlikely moments, when you're going about the business of your life, all wrapped up in something or someone that bears no relationship to your loss. It may be a word, a sight, a sound, a smell, a flitting memory. Suddenly the full impact of loss strikes you all over again. Hard.

Your grief is your own.

The same death will strike a dozen loved ones in a dozen different ways, each of them valid, each of them unique. The trick—and it really is unfair to call it a trick, since it's more a matter of luck and timing and perhaps the phase of the moon—is to be aware that grief is always lurking. Once you recognize that reality, you will be better equipped to beat it back into submission when you need to and to let it run its course when you're able.

In addressing a gathering of Gold Star family members who had lost loved ones in war, Vice President Joe Biden, whose wife and daughter died in an auto accident when he was 30, said: "There will come a day, I promise, when your thoughts of your son or daughter or husband or wife will bring a smile to your face before it brings a tear." He was right.

There's no deadline. You don't ever stop grieving someone you've loved, but you do eventually move on, as time quietly knits softer edges around the ragged hole left in your heart and your life.

If you are part of a support group for caregivers or related to your sibling's medical problem, those people can be tremendously helpful to you. Recognize, however, that what is happening to your family is not the happy ending that other participants may be envisioning. In fact, it may make some people extremely uncomfortable. Be prepared to lean elsewhere as well.

Grief counseling and support groups are widely available, and if your sibling was in hospice, those folks may have their own groups or be able to connect you with other local resources.

The Compassionate Friends is an international organization primarily devoted to parents who have lost children, but I attended sibling-related workshops at one of their national conferences and they have local chapters everywhere.

You are under no obligation to share anything, however, and if what you really want to do is just hole up by yourself, go right ahead and do it.

The American Cancer Society offers an excellent publication called "Coping with the Loss of a Loved One" that can be downloaded as a PDF from www.cancer.org. One issue addressed here is "complicated grief," defined as an extreme grief that continues for a prolonged period.

There's no good way to end a chapter about death, so I will let William Faulkner have the last word: "Between grief and nothing, I will take grief."

ADDITIONAL INFORMATION

Death

Mark Harris
Grave Matters: A Journey Through the Modern Funeral Industry to a Natural Way of Burial
Scribner, 2007

Melanie King
The Dying Game: A Curious History of Death
Portmeadow Books, 2012

Elisabeth Kubler-Ross
On Death and Dying
Touchstone, 1969

Elisabeth Kubler-Ross
Questions & Answers on Death and Dying
Touchstone, 1974

Jessica Mitford
The American Way of Death Revisited (published 1963, revised 1996)
Vintage, 2011

Sherwin B. Nuland
How We Die: Reflections of Life's Final Chapter
Vintage, 1995

End of Life

Jane Brody
Jane Brody's Guide to the Great Beyond
Random House, 2009

Katy Butler
Knocking on Heaven's Door: The Path to a Better Way of Life
Scriber, 2013

Ira Byock
The Best Care Possible: A Physician's Quest to Transform Care Through the End of Life
Avery, 2012

Joseph M. Champlin
Preparing for Eternity: A Catholic Handbook for End-of-Life Concerns
Ave Maria Press, 2007

David B. Feldman and S. Andrew Lasher, Jr.
The End-of-Life Handbook: A Compassionate Guide to Connecting with and Caring for a Dying Loved One
New Harbinger Publications, 2007

Jeanne Fitzpatrick and Eileen M. Fitzpatrick
A Better Way of Dying: How to Make the Best Choices at the End of Life
Penguin, 2010

Joyce Hutchinson and Joyce Rupp
May I Walk You Home? Courage and Comfort for Caregivers of the Very Ill, 10th Anniversary Edition
Ave Maria Press, 2009

David Kessler
The Needs of the Dying: A Guide for Bringing Hope, Comfort, and Love to Life's Final Chapter
Harper Perennial, 200

Joanne Lynn, Janice Lynch Schuster and Joan Harold
Handbook for Mortals: Guidance for People Facing Serious Illness, 2nd Edition
Oxford University Press, 2011

Dan Morhaim
The Better End: Surviving (and Dying) on Your Own Terms in Today's Medical World
Johns Hopkins University Press, 2011

Jo Myers
Good to Go: A Guide to Preparing for the End of Life
Sterling, 2010

Barbara Okun and Joseph Nowinski
Saying Goodbye: How Families Can Find Renewal Through Loss
Berkley, 2011

Felicity Warner
A Safe Journey Home: The Simple Guide to Achieving a Peaceful Death
Hay House, 2011

Bart Windrum
Notes from the Waiting Room: Managing a Loved One's End-of-Life Hospitalization
Axiom Action, 2008

Victoria Zackheim, ed.
Exit Laughing: How Humor Takes the Sting Out of Death
North Atlantic Books, 20120

Death of a Sibling

Elizabeth DeVita-Raeburn
Understanding Sibling Loss
Scribner, 2007

T.J. Wray
Surviving the Death of a Sibling
Three Rivers Press, 2003

P. Gill White
Sibling Grief: Healing After the Death of a Sister or Brother
iUniverse, 2008

Alan D. Wolfelt
Healing the Adult Sibling's Grieving Heart
Companion Press, 2008

Hospice

Hospice Foundation of America
www.hospicefoundation.org/
800.854.3402

Hospice Patients' Bill of Rights
Hospice Association of America
www3.nahc.org/haa/attachments/BillOfRights.pdf

National Hospice and Palliative Care Organization
www.caringinfo.org/
800.658.8898

National Hospice Foundation
www.nationalhospicefoundation.org
877.470.6472

• • • • •

Karen Whitley Bell
Living at the End of Life: A Hospice Nurse Addresses the Most Common Questions
Sterling Ethos, 2011

Maggie Callahan and Patricia Kelley
Final Gifts: Understanding the Special Awareness, Needs, and Communications of the Dying
Simon & Schuster reprint, 2012

Assisted Suicide

Compassion & Choices
(formerly The Hemlock Society)
www.compassionandchoices.org/

Final Exit Network
www.finalexitnetwork.org/

• • • • •

Derek Humphry
Final Exit: The Practicalities of Self-Deliverance and Assisted Suicide for the Dying, 3rd Edition
Delta Trade, 2002

Grief

American Cancer Society
Coping with the Loss of a Loved One
www.cancer.org

The Compassionate Friends
www.compassionatefriends.org

• • • • •

Pauline Boss
Ambiguous Loss: Learning to Live with Unresolved Grief
Harvard University Pressi, 1999

Allan Hugh Cole, Jr.
Good Mourning: Getting Through Your Grief
Westminster John Knox Press, 2008

Norine Dresser and Fredda Wasserman
Saying Goodbye to Someone You Love: Your Emotional Journey through End of Life and Grief
Demos Health, 2010

John W. James and Russell Friedman
The Grief Recovery Handbook, Twentieth Year Edition
William Morrow, 2009

ABOUT THE AUTHOR

Taffy Cannon is the author of fourteen published mysteries, an Academy Award-nominated short film, and *Convictions: A Novel of the Sixties*. As a *Jeopardy* contestant she once correctly wagered everything on a Women Writers Daily Double. She lives with her husband in Southern California, where she was named Citizen of the Year for service to her local library. Find out more at www.TaffyCannon.com

www.ingramcontent.com/pod-product-compliance
Lightning Source LLC
Chambersburg PA
CBHW070758280326
41934CB00012B/2960